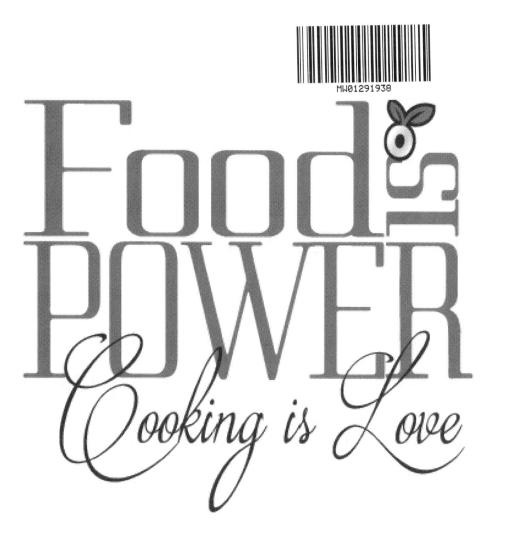

Food is POWER
Cooking is Love

How to make it Your wholesome meal

By Celebrity Chef Elisa Eliot

Food is Power, Cooking is love

How to Make it YOUR Wholesome Meal.

Cover Design, Illustrations & Layout by
Award Winning Designer Christina Michaelidis, owner of

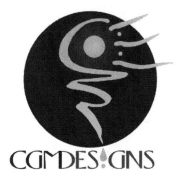

http://cgmdesigns.prosite.com
https://www.linkedin.com/in/christinamichaelidis
https://www.facebook.com/cgmdesigns/

This book is designed for educational purposes only and is not engaged in rendering medical advice, legal advice or professional services. If you feel that you have a medical problem, you should seek the advice of your Physician or health care Practitioner.

DEDICATION

What is your most important possession?

Your body.
You take IT everywhere you go and
It takes YOU everywhere you go.

Chef E

This book is dedicated to you, the one willing to participate in your health journey and wanting to know the truth about which foods can improve you and which foods can't. We live in a time when we have access to miraculous medicines, too. This book is for those who want both great food and great medicine.

I believe You are a magnificent, dynamic, physical, extension of God, the universe, the Divine. Let's eat like it. So, if you're privileged enough to have a home, then you are privileged enough to have home cooked meal.

This book is also dedicated to my greatest teacher, motivator, joy, and love. To my daughter Katie, "Have I told you lately, thanks for being my kid?"

TABLE OF CONTENTS

Ever been told your food's not love? I have, and they are right. Food is your power. Cooking is love. If you are confused by "wholesome" foods that have turned out not to be healthy in the long run and want to cut through the bull, then this book is for you. I cover a lot of ground. Some readers found following the outline really helped them.

FOREWORD

Dr. Kimmi Stultz, Clinical Pharmacist,
PharmD, Co-founder Juicery RX

As a clinical pharmacist, I learned from personal experience (having discovered I had an auto-immune disorder) that food has healing powers. Chef E understands the importance of food and the power that nutrients contribute to ensuring health and an overall mind, body, spirit sense of wellbeing.

Her knowledge from more than 30 years of experience and her sense of culinary adventure has taken her all over the world catering to everyone from celebrities, athletes and corporate executives to the extremely ill.

When I met Chef E, we had an instant synergy. She became immediately interested in my ideas of "prescribing" healthy food regimens that could work in tandem with traditional medications. Chef E began cooking and preparing meals for the people who had requested my assistance. Working together, we began to see that patients who started eating whole nutrient dense foods had a positive change in their physiology.

Her creative ideas, delicious and easy-to-create recipes, pantry lists, dining out tips, where to buy locally sourced organic produce, and how to navigate the grocery store as well as your own kitchen is like having a personal chef in your back pocket. Her book Food is Power is packed with valuable information and will become a trusted resource that not only will prove worthy in the kitchen, but will provide a go-to guide to living a healthier lifestyle, not only for yourself, but for your family.

Food can be a powerful form of medicine, it isn't just about calories in and calories out. Food contains information that communicates with our biology systems programming messages of health or illness. Your grocery store is your pharmacy; your kitchen is your medicine cabinet.

PREFACE

Ever hear the saying food's not love. They are right! Food is power. Cooking is love. You know that feeling when you invest yourself into feeding and nourishing someone you love? That's love. When you cook for some you love who is sick, or someone you love who has a big day tomorrow, well, that's when food is power.

This book has been simmering in me for a long time. It's taken me a while to process my experiences enough to share what I see that creates real success. These are my observations and verifiable solutions to overcome all-too-common problems for many people, like: "What's the right next step to improve my health? Where do I even begin? What do I eat? When can I feel better?"

I am so convinced of eating wholesome, in its truest definition of the word, that I started my own company called Wholesome Meal. Along with my nutritional chef work, I created and marketed a line of Snack Bites™ made from organic nut butters and brand name proteins. They are gluten-free and super portable and the perfect fix for those times you're traveling through the healthy food-barren places. Snack Bites™ are perfectly portioned and ideal for active, health-conscious individuals, and they are delicious! Quick, how many flavors of Snack Bites does it take to lose 80 pounds? Six, lol.

I wanted to call this book "Confessions of an Orthorexic Celebrity Catering Chef", but my editor talked me out of it. First of all, very few people have ever even heard of the term "Orthorexia" and if you Google it, you would find the following very negative definition:

"Orthorexia nervosa / ˌɔrθəˈrɛksiə nɜrˈvoʊsə/ (also known as orthorexia) is an eating disorder characterized by an extreme or excessive preoccupation with avoiding foods perceived to be unhealthy."

Seriously? Avoiding unhealthy foods is a disorder, a disease, a nervosa? Warning: Side effects include looking really hot, feeling really great, and having a lot of energy throughout the day. Please let me know when the pharmaceutical companies come out with a pill to cure me, because God knows I really want those 80 pounds I've lost back! I guess the only upside to this horrible disease is the worse your condition is, the better you look and feel. I just see something very wrong with our society if avoiding unhealthy foods labels someone as sick!

I want to make Wholesome Meal Snack Bites a huge success for my fellow Orthorexia Nervosa kindred spirits out there, as well as my new recruits to clean living. That's why Snack Bites are shipped directly to our stores and to our customers through our online stores and retailers. So there may be a few shameless plugs for Snack Bites in the book; *I just can't resist.*

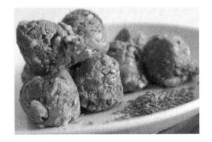

INTRODUCTION

Hello I'm Chef Elisa, but just call me Chef E. I'm an award winning, 5 star reviewed celebrity catering chef. I'm a catering chef beast. For more than 35 years I've been playing with fire, dry ice, knives and blow torches. My food is beyond ridiculous and I take no prisoners. When you come to one of my gigs you are mine. I don't care what diet you're on, it's a splurge night. You may come in the door strong, but by 2 appetizers into the evening and you're mine and you'll thank me too because my food passes the "worth the calories" test. Just check out my website www. chefelisascatering.com and verified reviews on Thumbtack, or my Facebook page and you see what I'm talking about. And... I'm also bi culinary. I cook naughty and nice.

What I learned from working one day week for celebs and sick folks took me **From this > To this**

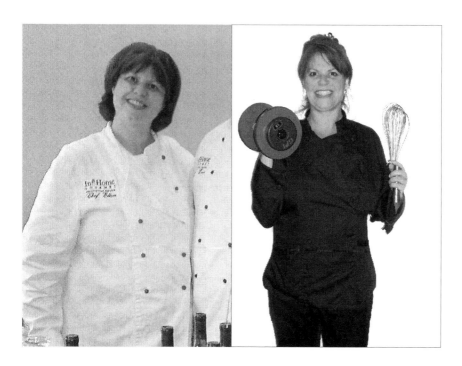

While cooking this…

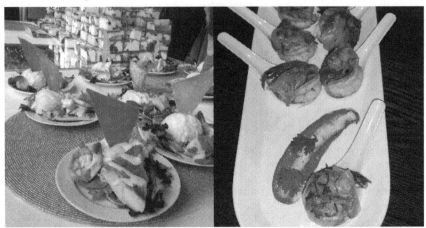

And eating this…

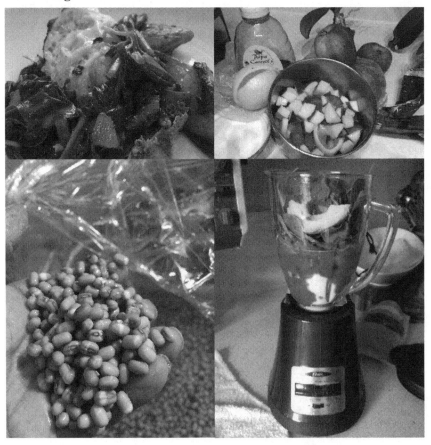

How does this happen? Welcome to my world.

For twenty years or so, every Monday, I have been cooking nutrition protocols I learned from cardiologists, cancer specialists, doctors, dieticians, gastroenterologists, medical centers, and many pro sports nutritionists. I took in all of their recommendations that worked and I discovered how to let the food assist in the healing. Whether the goal is for athletic endurance, weight loss, or healing from conditions such as diabetes, lung cancer, gut-lining cancer, brain function, tumors, heart disease and other various illnesses and stages of autoimmune diseases, I have assembled a Game Plan, a consensus of strategies from more than 100 nutrition protocols I learned from my experiences with high profile clients. I call it "a consensus of yeses", and it's the cornerstone of my Play Book for *your healing* plan.

I have had the privilege to cook for Ata and Dwayne Johnson, Dan Marino and his family, Former Miami Dolphin's General Manager Jeff Ireland's daughters', actor Tommy Lee Jones's family, Former NFL players Jason Taylor, Terry, Kirby, Chris GrAtan, NHL Florida Panther hockey players, The Indigo Girls, heavyweight champion Shannon Briggs, Walt Freese, former CEO for Stony Brook Farms and Ben & Jerry's, Dr. Burton Grossman, Texas Billionaire philanthropist, Adam Terris, minor league baseball player and clients of Dr. Bret Emery, Behavioral Medicine, including Atlanta Braves baseball players, professional golfers, members of Lance Armstrong's U.S. Cycling Team, Good Taste TV's and former television news anchor Tanji Patton, WWE professional wrestler Sarona Tamina Snuka and close to a hundred more clients each with specific dietary needs.

Wholesome [hohl-suh m] - adjective 1. conductive to bodily health; healthful; beneficial 2. suggestive of physical health, especially in appearance.

I believe words having specific definitions and meanings. So when I say Wholesome, I mean conducive your body's health. This book is intended to help you update way the way you evaluate, shop, cook, and eat the foods that are right for you.

I have learned a great deal from my clients and my own experiences, and now I want to share all of that with you to create your own game plan for success. Ready? Read on!

PS – I write like I speak, which is with high-energy, humor, slang, and LOTS of passion!

This book covers a lot of info, so following the outline is very helpful. ☺

CHAPTER ONE - 2016 QUICK FOOD UPDATE

(Snap. Snap. Snap) Hey, it's okay. You're okay. Look, while you were in the wheat brain, sugar gut fog, a few things changed: shag carpet is back, shoulder pads are out, and pants are still skinny for guys and girls. I'm so sorry and glad at the same time that you are gluten intolerant now, but it doesn't have to be forever. Maybe no one has told you yet, but if you are gluten intolerant, then you absolutely ARE sugar intolerant. I know, I know, you don't want to hear it, but I know where Sugar Freedom is, and you can live there or just visit from time to time; it's your choice.

I have some big assists; game changers I've learned from serving ridiculously successful clients. For 20 years or so, I have been cooking nutrition protocols I learned from cardiologists, cancer specialists, dieticians, gastroenterologists, and sports nutritionists. I learned how to let the food help you. I've cooked for Ata Johnson and Dwayne Johnson, Texas billionaire Dr. Burton Grossman and a bunch more pro athletes, sick folks, and body builders. I can tell you it's a new game with new rules now. You woke up so that proves you have what it takes to heal, so now you just need to find the foods that fix you. And bonus: I learned how to make some dope food, too, so you won't even miss the convenient chemistry experiments you ate from the drive thru!

Now some of what I'm about to tell you may freak you out, but I want you to know it's going to be okay and it's getting better already. The science is improving and the new economic growth is in the green industries that are looking for ways to minimize our toxic risks. Organic sales are the only growth area in the food biz and soda sales are down as well as cereal sales. In fact, every time you buy something organic, the market responds by making more organic products. The global science is, for the first time ever, available for global public consumption and we're all learning a lot from each other.

In keeping with full disclosure, I think it's important for you know I'm a big fan of western medicine. I don't see an either-or between great nutrition and great medicine. It was in one of my early experiences of cooking for billionaire philanthropist Dr. Burton Grossman where I learned how great nutrition's goal IS to remove obstacles to healing. I first called this "clearing the deck for the docs". Now I like to think of it as "creating the space for success".

Ok, so it's a new game.
The game has gone global and there are a few news rules.

Here's your overview: In the last 60 years, physicians, industrial products, and foods & drug manufactures have introduced hundreds and hundreds of new chemicals into us annually. There are now over 84,000 chemicals in our "stuff" today, and according to the Environmental Protection Agency (EPA), only 200 have been tested. Jim Jones, the Assistant Administrator of the EPA in a recent interview said, "The EPA cannot assure the American consumer of a product's safety". So here's Rule #1: Don't assume it's safe, **our laws are not constructed that way.**

According to the movie "Food Inc.", more than 3,000 chemicals are in our food and the average processed meal contains 1,500 to 1,800. It's likely more today, since Food Inc. was made in 2009. The vast majority of the additives, fillers, and chemicals are FDA classified as GRAS: generally recognized as safe. But several of the GRAS chemicals are not allowed in Europe as they are in the American food market place. Since there are so many and I honestly I can't remember the vast majority of the names of the chemicals, additives and preservatives. I just call them "all that jazz". Preservatives I typically refer to as "Pixie Dust", because the food never grows old.

Likely the most controversial foods on the market contain GMOs, genetically modified organisms. GMO grains were approved for animal feed in 1988 and introduced to the US food supply by 1996. The patented genetic modifications include a resistance to their proprietary pesticide glyphosate; the plant produces its own pesticide through its proteins so when a bug tries to eat it, its gut explodes. (Yes, it does sound a lot like what's happening to you too). And finally, a "suicide gene" is embedded, so the plant dies before it reseeds itself, forcing the farmers to purchase new seed every year.

On March 23, 2015 The World Health Organization declared the pesticide glyphosate a "probable human carcinogen" and is actively encouraging more studies. And over the years here in the US, repeated political and legal attempts have been made to protect GM companies from legal action by installing language into bills to construct pre-emption, or pre-empt the state's and consumer's rights to litigate. The industries are also fighting hard to keep us in the dark and fighting labeling efforts here and in other countries. The GM companies have farms all over the world now, so lots of us are eating them with some countries labeling them, like Russia, China and Europe. Just not us.

But for now, we have to play the I Spy game to find them. (I've got a secret decoder ring for you later.) These crops are primarily, corn, soy, and canola. GMO corn isn't just used for corn products such as corn starch, baking soda, corn oil, and syrup; in fact, many preservatives and vitamins, including citric acid, are also derived from it. Sugar beets, zucchini, and cotton are on the market and more GMO crops are on their way; salmon, apples, and potatoes have been approved by the FDA.

As far as this global game goes… well, I'm just not sure we should be putting the pieces in our mouths just yet. I think we need some more studies and time. The latest bill our government is pushing hard for, as of writing this, is a trade deal called Trans Pacific Partnership that would eliminate

COOL (Country of Origin Labeling) and open the door to outsourcing the processing of our poultry to China. This would further encourage US poultry manufacturers to outsource the butchering and processing as well as the battering, breading, and seasoning processes to China. China does not have the same inspection systems in place that we enjoy in this country, so it's definitely something you want to be aware of with everything you buy.

Do you know why the people in China wear the face masks? So they can cross the street and get to the other side. It's not so much the bird flu, the substandard inspections, or business practices; it's the pollution.

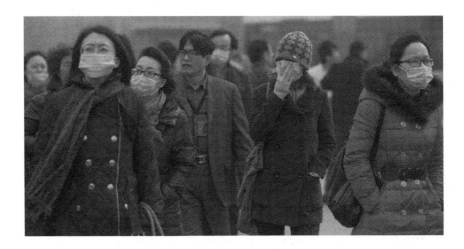

China's pollution levels are more than seven times above the World Health Organization's recommended maximum. The pollution from producing plastics, our gadgets, gizmos, and rare earth minerals is driving the pollution production and political unrest. And speaking of driving, in January 2014 an ABC news reporter clocked 450 miles outside Beijing before he could see the sun past the pollution. These pollution impacts are based on which way the wind blows, too. And remember the nuclear melt down at Fukushima? Notice how everyone still has their lights on even though they don't have nuclear power? Nice trick, right? They are back to burning coal, so hello to mercury and all that that brings to the seafood industry. And speaking of seafood, according to a Bloomberg report 27 percent of the seafood we Americans eat comes from China, the book American Catch quotes 88% from Asia in general is consumed in the US and the FDA inspects only 2.7% of imported food. So…. the whole, "fish is healthy" thing, I'm not so sure about for the moment.

And here's what's happening to us.

During the same years that GMOs were quietly being introduced into animal and human food, other new industries such as plastics, fire retardants, materials for clothing, toys, anti-depressants and cosmetic technologies were also rapidly growing. Then beginning in 1988, childhood cancer rates, obesity rates, infertility, and allergy rates have all seen dramatic upticks in numbers of incidents. Our children and our ability to make them have been impacted and challenged by our collective exposures. In 1999 about the same time peanut butter got banned from the school lunch space, a new word became part of our collective vocabulary, is Autism. As of the 2014 CDC report, it's now 1 in 68. If this statistical trend continues 1 in 2 will be born with autism in just ten more years. Yes, you heard me right, I said half of our children will be born autistic in 2025. This alarming increase in gut break down starting with IBS has also given rise to a whole new category pharmaceutical drugs to sell.

Unraveling this tangled ball of new technology and chemical introductions will likely be a complex, litigious, and lengthy process. You don't have to wait for them to clean up this mess. There is a way to navigate the "all that jazz" to start feeling better, and I have a fun way to start. We're going to go through the process I use for my clients to get your nutrition AND fridge geared up for you.

Oh but wait, I know you're not just thinking about yourself; you're thinking of your loved ones, too. It's ok, it's just food! That's what I'll show you how to play with. The stuff that, in the famous words of Groucho Marx, couldn't Hoyt. That's food. And once you prepare your base foods, or in Chef talk, your "mise en place" (which is a really fancy French way of saying you have your sh*% together), the rest is easy. Everyone will be able to pull what they need from your fridge.

Psssst, here's a clue, if food were supposed to be complicated, we all would have perished a millennium ago. Trust me, this is cake... okay not cake, but it's very easy. Oh, and speaking of cake... I'm a firm believer in the weekly splurge meal or two. I will share ways to minimize that impact too.

Here are my Quick Clues for you.
Don't eat controversy or secrets.
Look for a legit consensus of yeses!
Buy the change you want to be.

CHAPTER TWO - HOW WE ABSORB NUTRIENTS

Over View: Understanding your physical game and how to connect with the right food for you

In this game your body is pre-programmed for Do-Overs, Resets and Counter-Measures. These preprogrammed, autocorrect systems are your healing and renewal cellular processes. You constantly slough off dead cells, skin, hair, uterine lining, gut tissue, the whole body. Different organs and tissues renew at different rates. Current science estimates uterine tissue re-sets monthly. New gut and intestinal tissue is revealed on a five-day schedule and what you eat today is the skin you wear in 30 days. You are growing a "new you" all the time. You have a complex and beast immune system I'll explain as The D Triple G & the F R B.

Current medical science tells us 85% of illness stems from nutrient deficiency. So, for example, Ricketts stems from a Vitamin D deficiency, Scurvy stems from a Vitamin C deficiency and depression is linked to magnesium, omega 3's and Vitamin D.

Ever since I caught on fire, I know what nutrients make skin. I know, a hell of way to learn something. But hey, it stuck and so did my skin graft with a 98% adhesion rate, which is pretty good since as skin grafts go. Anything above 35% percent is considered a success.

So tissue is made up of proteins, essential amino acids, and Vitamins A, C, and E, and zinc. Our bodies recycle and even manufacture some of these nutrients, but we don't make the "essential amino acids". We have to eat them. There are 17 vitamins, 12 minerals, and 5 trace minerals; and when we don't have all or some of the them, we become ill. In fact, it's estimated that 85% of all chronic illnesses are caused by nutrient deficiencies. Research that shows links between vitamin C deficiency and scurvy, vitamin

D deficiencies with rickets and cancer, and so on. That way, doctors agree, pharmacists agree, and everyone agrees. **We have a consensus of yeses!**

Where do you find these nutrients? **We have a consensus of yeses here too**. Food! Ding ding ding! It's so powerful that it's where big pharma is looking to develop their components. 'Food First' is Life Extension's motto. My friends food has triple points in this game!

Food is a 3'fer

1. It instantly energizes and nourishes.
2. It forms and becomes us: our tissue, our muscles, our skin.
3. It detoxes our self-cleaning system by aiding in the removal what we don't need.

Let's start at First Base: Absorption

So how exactly how do we absorb the vitamins, minerals, and nutrients? Well here's my super basic explanation: your stomach muscles contract and churn enzymes from the food you ate, along with the digestive juices and enzymes you bring to the party, compliments of your gallbladder. The solid foods are smooshed into a liquid mixture, basically. Our gut-lining tissues act like sponges to then absorb them and then use them for a good night's work of creating new tissue, muscle, skin, bone, brain, and everything. Talk about you really are what you eat! Here's a link to tummy in action, taken by doctors at Massachusetts General Hospital.

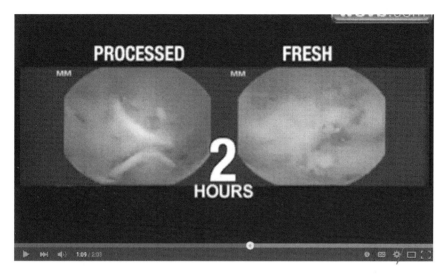

www.youtube.com/watch?v=IQlNv2Au-Lg

This very cool video, shot with a camera pill, shows how the gut contracts and churns to smoosh everything into mush to be absorbed. The tummy on the left has the instant ramen noodles from the grocery store and the one on the right has fresh noodles prepared at a local restaurant. The differences are the fresh noodles didn't contain preservatives, nor were they micro-waved and cooked in plastic as you're instructed to do, so a lot more factors are in play with the packaged version from the grocery. You will notice these doctors can't legally say preservatives challenge nutrition upload, but it's kind of clear that when the noodles didn't become mushy after two hours and the fresh noodles became smoosh within twenty minutes… that something's different. That's a clue. Since our gut linings absorb the smoosh mush as it moves through our tissues, kind of like water through a sponge, it doesn't take a brain surgeon to see the video shows that's not happening with the dried noodles. And now many recent studies are linking compromised gut-lining tissue with compromised nutrition absorption, as we learn more about autism, fragile gut linings, and illness.

That's when I caught a big clue: it's just not enough to eat the nutrient-dense foods; we also need to absorb them, and fats in your food are super beneficial for nutrition absorption. The fats are how fat-soluble vitamins A, D, E, and K are uploaded, such as how non-fat soluble vitamins hitch a ride. Nutrient absorption is still a big mystery, but we do know the nutrients specifically in an apple, tomato, or in dairy are interconnected and dependent upon each other for absorption. Calcium is a great example of this. You don't absorb the calcium unless vitamin D is on board and vitamin D requires vitamins K1 and K2 to unlock and so on and so on and so on. We have a 3-hour opportunity to absorb the nutrition of what we eat or experience inflammation.

Inflammation is actually a very good thing. Yes, it's defined as reddened, swollen, hot, and irritated tissue; it's actually the body's first line of defense. So let's say you accidentally take a sip of a beverage you realize your sick child just slobbered all over. Well then, inflammation is exactly what you need at that moment. When the gut tissue is swollen, the cells constrict; it minimizes what gets through and stops the threat from going any farther into our body's system.

However, if you're eating or breathing something on a consistent schedule and firing off your inflammatory response, then that's when it's bad thing. Kind of like crying wolf, but unlike getting ignored it's the exact opposite. Your body gets super confused and thinks it itself is the threat and it Atacks. There is a progression that diseases take: inflammatory conditions left unresolved get bigger and become conditions classified as autoimmune conditions, which include arthritis, psoriasis, and Crohn's disease. The problem is, when autoimmune doesn't get rolled back, it often transitions into cancer. So the takeaway here is inflammation is a very good thing; it's just less is more, because chronic inflammation begets autoimmune, and autoimmune begets cancer.

CHAPTER THREE - FEELING BETTER IS BIG

Having cooked briefly for Former Dolphins General Manager, Jeff Ireland's daughters who have celiac and autism, learning about how leaky gut syndrome impacts nutrient deficiency made perfect sense to me. Since to me it's first base; everything starts from here. Nurturing their fragile and shredded gut linings best as possible was the focus. In these experiences, the clients and I know the nutrients are going in, but we needed to understand how to create the best opportunities for them upload and minimize the inflammatory response.

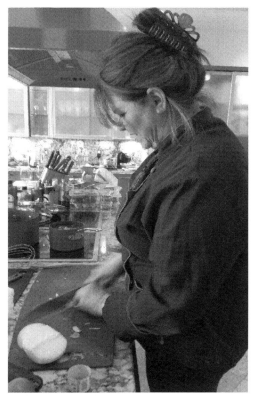

In the summer of 2013, I took on a client who had peritoneal mesothelioma, which is cancer of the gut lining. The first day I met with Jennybeth, I walked in to find her loving husband preparing her a gluten-free waffle swimming i n maple syrup. You see, Jennybeth was quickly losing weight so, in desperate search for calories, they turned to sugar. I was clearly alarmed to see this, and here's the part where I lose my mind every time I think of it: no other health care professional in her hundreds and hundreds of appointments since her early development of IBS more than 35 years ago, nor any physician on her current cancer team (this being her second round of Peritoneal mesothelioma of the gut lining cancer) ever, and I do mean ever, communicated how sugar was proven to dissolve gut lining tissue. Not one! I was THE first to explain how sugar was challenging her gut, her tissues, and her life. I was also the first to prove it to her. The doctor who referred her to me called me about two weeks into our work and shared with me the unexpected news that made me cry tears of joy. Jennybeth started having "normal" bowel movement seven days into her wholesome meal program. It was amazing to witness her body respond so well. Her nutrient levels were checked every 30 to 60 days, so when her iron dropped, I was able to adjust her diet with foods rich in iron, and then watch her levels return to "her normal" levels.

My job was to help her keep weight on and keep her iron levels in a good range. What was interesting to learn was at times her iron levels would drop, even though her diet was consistent. I learned how to view this perspective, since a drop was a precursor for her health worsening. So then it became a situation where we increased her intake of iron-rich foods and looked for other factors that would diminish her absorption. And the first place to look is for inflammation, the first obstacle to nutrition absorption. Inflammation presents itself often as red, swollen, and irritated tissue. In very basic terms, our bodies produce this immune reaction when something comes in it perceives as a threat. So when the gut tissue is swollen, the cells constrict, minimizing what gets through and stopping the threat from going any farther into our body's system.

The story of my lovely Jennybeth ended about a year into our journey. Jnnybeth had already done the gut chemo treatments once before and they gave her another five years of life. But she really didn't want to do it again. That journey was very difficult; it almost killed her. Instead she chose to explore non-conventional treatments for a while.

During our year she felt so much better that she went to some parties, loved on her granddaughters, and even got in a game or two of tennis with her husband, but she also knew she was fighting for her quality of life. When the non-conventional treatments failed her, she chose to pursue chemo treatments again. She was afraid, but she was strong and we had a liquid food plan she could freeze and ship. When her surgeons opened her up and inserted the chemo pack into her gut lining, only then did they see her lining was so badly broken down. This was something they did not expect, given her current weight and how well she was functioning. She died the next day… in peace. So even if her food didn't fix her, it sure made her function and feel better for the last year of life. And that alone is so huge it brings me to tears every time I think about it; it's a priceless, enormous gift.

My many clients suffering with fragile gut linings gave me insights into some processes behind the labels that can trigger inflammation. I'm going to talk more fully about these in the chapter 'Evaluate the 3 P's: Preservatives, Pesticides, and Processes.'

CHAPTER FOUR - YOUR IMMUNE SYSTEM

Our bodies are in the constant process of absorbing 2016 technology through a world of new flavors, products, and chemicals from literally all over the world. And understanding how we can assist our own body's built-in autocorrect is extremely helpful. I call this butt saving trick 'The D, Triple G and the F, R, B'.

The D, triple G, The D, triple G, The D, triple G and the F, R, B
It's got a good beat, I can dance to it, I'll give it 10!

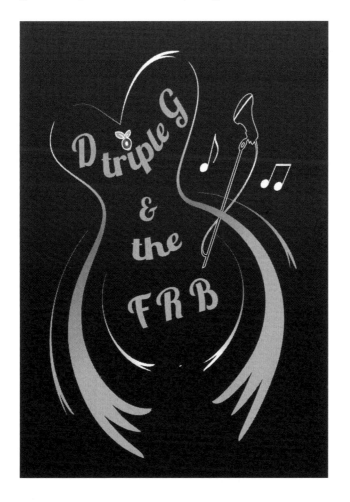

The D stands for Don't come in. That's inflammation, reddened, swollen, hot, and often painful tissues, which we just covered in the previous chapter.

The triple G part is get out, get out, get out

Which happens how? Through your pee, poop, and sweat.

The first G is for tinkling. Going often enough is essential to removing toxins. Staying hydrated is the fix. Most doctors agree your urine should run clear. Now that's great info for guys… but for us girls, our visual indicator is, let's say, diluted. So when the toilet bowl water is orange, please know the actual concentration is much darker. Frequent urination is a good thing. It's telling you your body's self-cleaning systems are flowing strong.

The Second G is Poop. Ready for the straight poop on pooping? It takes approximate three hours for our foods to fully digest. I learned this from Dr. Brett Emery along with many other sports trainers. So that's why athletes will time how long it takes to poop after eating. ☺ Just sharing.
Fun Fact Did you know top athletes can poop 5 times a day?

Doctors agree you should be pooping at least once a day. Once you get your hydration set, this usually "autocorrects". By 30 to 60 days, most clients begin to poop twice a day. My more constipated and dehydrated clients find making their own chia seed drinks at night before bed is super helpful.

A great drink is 1 tablespoon seeds + 6 to 8 ounces of water + a squeeze or muddle of fruit such as berries, melon, or lemon, or even muddled cucumber. Chia seeds only need about 5 to 6 hours to fully hydrate but will patiently wait for you for up to 12 hours. After 24 hours, juicing aficionados agree the mojo and nutrient value is dramatically reduced without preserving.

You really shouldn't have a great need for toilet paper. I knew things were getting messy when I saw the grocery aisle expand with wipes for adults.

In fact, it's usually a nice big surprise for my clients when things start working out so smoothly. Tracking how well you poop is a big clue to identifying your power foods.

The third G is Sweat. Sweat not only regulates your body's temperature, it purges toxins from your system. Sweating is even better when my heart rate is up there and I feel the sweat dripping down my back and my breath is so strong and deep. Yah! I'm talking about working-out. And if you were thinking naughty thoughts then whoa, soldier! That's another sign your body is ready for some healing, so get your booty to the gym.

Exercise is a big deal to detoxing the body. Even just 20 minutes of cardio everyday will pay off big. Now if you're like me, starting out as a pure novice with some weakness, balance, and health stuff going on... then find a good trainer. Even if only for a couple of months. A good trainer will teach you how to get comfortable in the gym. They should give you hand-outs and custom workouts for you to keep.

Find a way, make it happen; it's that important. As a single mom and chef entrepreneur, I could not afford these services, so I found a way. Hint: some trainers will work for food— good food, that is. In business it's called bartering and it's how I have been able to afford a trainer twice weekly and a massage therapist weekly for most of my personal journey. Trust me, these two pieces are critical for my solution.

Tips for bartering: find mom and pop gyms and spas. The trainers and therapists usually have more autonomy vs. working at a franchise. Find a good trainer, do your homework, and put out requests on www.Thumbtack. com or other lead services to get a connect. Cook for them at the same time you cook for yourself. You'll be able to streamline your time better and offer your barter more variety. I base mine on my hourly rate of $75 per hour against theirs. So if I'm getting two hours, I'll put in about $30 in food cost and the rest in my time for a service that would cost $140.00. When you drop their production inside your own, the extra time you may choose to invest will be invested into you as well.

My trainer is Gareth Ross, American College of Sports Medicine CPT, Personal Training Director and Tactical Athlete Program Director at Ultimate Sports Institute. He is one of the best I have ever had. I'm feeling great and get stronger each day; I'm in the best physical condition ever. We don't do crazy jumpy cardio climbing stuff or anything else that will jeopardize my need to have my legs and back intact to be the badass catering chef that I am. We do something called sports medicine-based fitness, which improves my strength, balance, and ultimately my catering chef performance. Functional movement and training is another way to explain this.

I asked Gary what are the top three benefits to working out that he saw his clients get and here's what he said:

• Resolution of pain or discomfort

• Increased and renewed self-esteem and confidence

• Feeling of empowerment

You weren't expecting that, were you? Neither was I when I asked, but damn if it's not true! And notice, even though losing body fat is also happening, it didn't make his top three. There are even better "game changing" rewards in play. Weight loss is the byproduct of the other body systems coming in line.

He got me out of ridiculous daily pain in under 30 days. In a few months, I was feeling beast, so it's showed in my career; and since I learned the moves to stretch, foam roll, and activate my body, I am empowered with the knowledge of how to keep what I have achieved. Trust me you'll want to Youtube or google it for the correct moves for you. I start my day from the ground up.

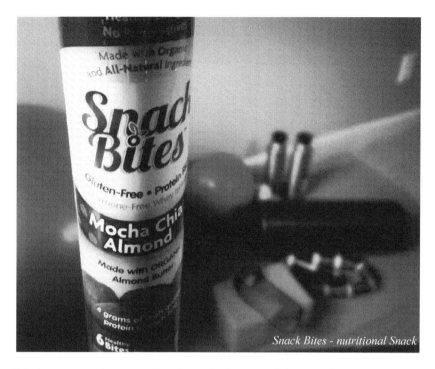

Snack Bites - nutritional Snack

This is my stretch space. I rock my body a good three to four times a week on gigs that run 18 hours. I also have a small fracture on my L5 vertebra. Keeping my muscles intact and in the right place is key for me, and it's vital for my career. I warm up my legs and back with a heating pad while meditating and then I stretch before I jump into my day. Heating the muscles before stretching with light activity, dynamic stretching or with a heating pad is super important.

Stretching, muscle contractions, and blood flow all reduce body inflammation and pain if done correctly. Stretching movements need to be repeated 6 to 8 times and held for at least 10 seconds. I am a Foam rolling fool. It is a huge help and when you foam roll you need to stay on the spot that is tight and hurts for about a minute to gain the full benefit of the myofascial release. You control how much pressure you permit during foam rolling. I am now able to get out of significant levels of pain without pain relievers and anti-inflammatory medications. This is part of my Daily Diligence.

A sports deep-tissue massage is a game changer as you rebuild your body. Now the reason this section is under sweat is this style of massage is physically intense and often a dance between that sensation between intense pain then relief, all tickly and warm. In my case, there is a fair amount of grunting and I make noises I've never even heard before. You see, she is pushing out the clotted blood and lactic acid, smoothing muscle tissue, pulling on ligaments, and generally putting muscles back where they belong. If I didn't have this in place, I am positive I wouldn't have had the ability to push harder. Relieving discomfort is a big key! Thumbtack, LinkedIn, and other leads services are great ways to connect with barter opportunities.

And the F, R, B!

F stands for fat. Fat plays a big role in protecting the body from threats and starvation. The ability to create fat cells to store extra vitamins and calories for times of famine or sickness is an awesome trick. Fat cells are also created to store the toxins you take in, to protect the body from them just wandering around inside you. While reading Sweet Deception by Dr. Mercola, I learned our bodies will create fat cells to encase "foreign" matter as a part of our own autoimmune response system. That's why doctors are finding new compositions of fat cells, which are alive and apparently transmitting estrogen signals. Yah, I can't make this stuff up.

So what's in your fat cells? Well, if losing weight is a first on, last off game, then mine are vintage 1970 Jiffy Pop ᵗᵐ, Fiddle Faddle ᵗᵐ, boil in bag chili mac, red M & M's ᵗᵐ and Do Dads ᵗᵐ chased with orange Nehi ᵗᵐ soda pop! So when I burn the fat in that cell, I am what… re-releasing the contents, whether toxic or nutritious, into my system. Now that you know this, let's say we roll back the idea of rapid weight loss and chug a thermos of water! The 1 to 2 pound per week rule is a good one. Rapid weights loss risks include losing your gall bladder, which then compromises your ability to metabolize fats from your food.

Fun Fact Plants and animals respond in kind. Fat cells store goodies and toxins; so buy the best fats you can afford.

R is for restore which includes meditation.

Sleep is when you fix. It's one of only two times your body releases growth hormones. Neuroscience explains that when we think we're doing nothing, the polar opposite is true. Our brains are flushing fluids to clear out debris, our tissues are restoring, and healing happens. Remember how food is a 3fer? Well, Part 2 is here. Those 17 vitamins, 12 minerals, and 5 trace minerals are becoming your skin on the inside and a lot of this work is done while you sleep. Don't feel guilty if you need more sleep than the others. If you're not getting enough sleep, find a way to get it! Don't deprive yourself the opportunity to heal. Naps are great! Athletes love them and most do it daily! Latest neuroscience shows 9 hours is better than 8 hours; and if your activity is healing, the more the merrier.

Meditation restores and reboots your brain waves and is proven to increase your melatonin levels improving your sleep as well so you require less. I personally went from typically needing 10 to 11 hours daily down to 9 and some days less. I didn't know how or what meditation was when I first started, so I love the Oprah and Deepak 21-day Guided Meditation series. You can sample them for free online.

I like to "namastay in bed" first thing in the am and meditate while I heal my adrenals. I don't feel guilty about sleeping extra because I'm mediating ;-) ;-) . I wake up and drink some green tea from a thermos on my nightstand that I made the night before. So I'm uploading a little caffeine, staying PH neutral, and meditating! This is my happy place. Welcome.

B is for Breath. Are you taking deep breaths right now or short shallow breaths? Funny thing about deep breaths: they sure do help me feel better, emotionally and physically. Ever notice a weight lifter take in really deep breaths before doing the lift? Even Tony Robbins has a whole breathing routine every morning to fully activate his physicality. Breath and oxygen levels are translated into energy. Breathing in oxygen is essential in detoxifying your cells. Oxygen's (negative electrical charge) Ataches itself to the toxins in the cells and neutralizes their positive charge. Cell impurities become less magnetic and therefore less toxic and easier for the body to remove. Being short on oxygen is no joke either. When we go to the doctor, they often clip a piece of equipment on our finger called a pulse oximeter. It gives them a general idea of how much oxygen is in our blood. And your brain is the hog. The brain uses about three times as much oxygen as muscles in the body do. So everything from alertness to mood are impacted.

When I consulted with heavyweight champion Shannon "The Cannon" Briggs who, in his own words, is a "freak of nature", I learned this dude has asthma. Yah. Avoiding foods that cause congestion and enhancing his lung performance is critical to his career. So it was a little Jewish penicillin to the rescue or, in today's lingo, bone broth. Dr. Stephen Rennard, a pulmonary expert at the University of Nebraska Medical Center in Omaha, found evidence the soup contains anti-inflammatory properties, which is why it helps when we get a cold. It's such a health bonus that I have it in our Wholesome Meal Game Plan.

CHAPTER FIVE - COOKING FOR DR. GROSSMAN

How I got here to this culinary space

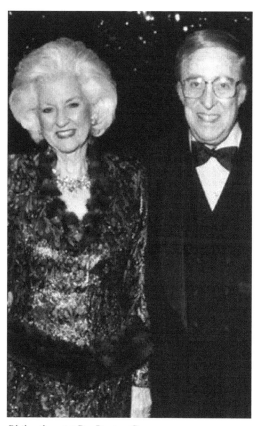

Philanthropist Dr. Burton Grossman

The Wholesome standard first came into being in 1998 in San Antonio Texas with client Billionaire Philanthropist Dr. Burton Grossman. I had a few years of cooking various diets under my belt when I got the call to interview for the job. I had great success with several type 2 diabetes/weight loss clients and a triple heart bypass client who after only three months on the Dallas Cooper Clinic diet was able to reduce his blood pressure medications to resume his extra-curricular activities with his mistress ;-) ;-). (Yes, some folks do tell the chef TMI. But I digress).

I was confident I could have good results with Dr. Grossman. Meeting him was pretty exciting. He lived the in the most exclusive penthouse property in San Antonio, Texas. I first saw him when as he was getting into his glass cylinder-shaped elevator inside his penthouse, which was quiet and smooth as silk as it delivered him from the second floor to the first. He was insanely rich, old, and charming. He was just a good ole Texan who just wanted some southern comfort food his doctors would OK. So when he told me he'd be my "best friend" if I made him some biscuits and gravy, I almost wet my pants; I was so excited. I had this! I was an expert at cooking by the numbers by now. It was 1998, the era of low-fat everything, artificial sweeteners, artificial flavors, and MSG. I was set!

His European physicians gave me a type one diabetes/ heart disease blended protocol to follow. The goal set was this: his diet was to keep his sugar levels stable. Now these were tall orders (even in Texas) for any chef. So I measured and calculated every ingredient I used to create accurate protein, carbohydrate, fat, and calories counts for every meal I cooked.

So you know what I did next? Yep, I sure did. Biscuits and Gravy, made from low-fat this, powdered that and frozen breakfast styled turkey sausage patties all jacked up on GMO preservatives and stabilizers, MSG artificial flavors and low fat! I popped a little steamed broccoli and asparagus on the plate for good measure and voila! Biscuits and Gravy all within in his calories, fat, protein, and carbs. Tadahhhh! Now instead of getting a new super-rich BFF, my phone rang and I heard frantic voices on the other end asking, "What did you feed him?? What did you feed him? His sugars are at 280." It was not a good day to be me.

Dr. Grossman had a number of other health conditions in play simultaneously, so hitting the mark was a bit of moving target. The stress of being sick, family, and business matters to attend to and numerically correct but chemically jacked up diet (I realize now) created havoc with his blood sugars.

Moving forward, his physicians requested photocopies of every food label of every ingredient that I was using for Dr. Grossman's menu. I was to wait for the OK to make his meal, which I did. While Dr. Grossman's meal contained calories, protein, fats, and carbohydrate numbers that were right on point and doctor approved, that didn't matter. Who knows which ingre-dient or ingredients caused the inflammation and elevated sugar counts to almost 300? All I knew was, by the third episode, I found myself fired and minus my new philanthropist bff. His doctors insisted he move to Europe to continue his care there.

What I know now that I didn't know then is there are more studies than I can say grace over that link inflammation to elevated blood sugars, acidic body chemistry, gut imbalance, arthritis and heart disease.

The lesson here is to evaluate the content and the composition of the calorie. And if you can't, then when in doubt, leave it out.

CHAPTER SIX – EVALUATE THE 3 P'S

This Your Secret Decoder Ring to evaluating the content and the composition of the calorie. Evaluate it, don't judge it. Evaluate as best you can the 3 p's: pesticides, preservatives and processes, looking for preservative technology they may not be on the label.

Quick Clue: Don't eat controversy or secrets. Companies have never been more accessible or open to answering customer questions than now. Got a question? Tweek it and tag the manufacturer, ask on their FaceBook page, hit them up on Instagram or send then an email if your question is complex. ***It's easy peasy!***

Preservatives. Here are the main two things I want to explain about preservatives, organic, conventional or artificial:

1. They alter the original enzyme content of the food to prevent breakdown. Our gall bladders and pancreas provide only part of the digestive enzymes required to breakdown foods and absorb the nutrients; the other part comes from the food. If we take that away, what does that do? How do we offset that impact? And while you saw the Noodle video, some preservatives do a lot more. So as I focus on the uploading part of the nutrition equation, my first goal is to avoid anything that can compromise absorption.

2. The vast majority of preservatives on the market work like this: they increase the acidity of the food in the jar, the bottle, the can, the sippy bag or box to prevent spoilage. Often the foods in the jar, bottle, can, sippy bag or box start out alkaline or are served over food that is alkaline, such as your salad. In so shifting the natural balance of your meal from alkaline to acidic. As you can see from this chart, almost all of your fruits and veggies are alkaline to PH neutral. So lemon, lettuce, tomato, cucumber, and olive

oil are all alkaline and are intended to be alkaline. But instead you are now pouring a salad dressing or sauce with preservatives on it and now this is shifting the PH of the meal more toward acidic.

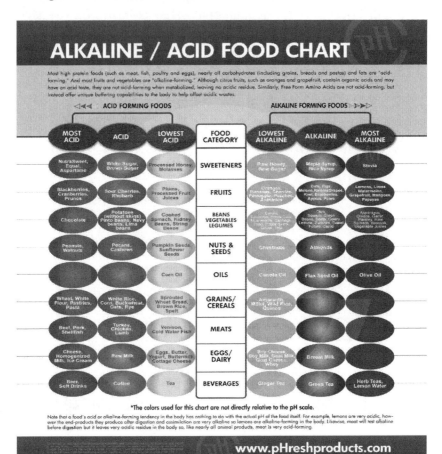

The convenience food industry depends on these preservatives to create the time for them to get their products through the matrix. So now virtually everything you eat has a higher acidity level than originally intended. And for those whose lives have been touched by cancer, these words resonate for a reason. Acidity and cancer go hand in hand. Keeping meals' indigenous PH levels truly has served me well. That's why we'll make our own dressings, fruit sauces, and condiments.

So one day my lovely child asked me to make a meal she had a friend's house that she just loved. This meal required Wish Bone ᵗᵐ Italian dressing. But as any torn mother would do, I begrudgingly said yes. I marinated 2 pounds of organic chicken in this concoction for the week. I used about a pound that weekend with friends and left the rest to marinate. This bag of marinating chicken fell to the back of the fridge which I discovered about 2 weeks later. I don't know why, maybe the chef thing, maybe the Italian thing, but I sniffed it. And, surprise, it smelled fine. So I kept it and continued the experiment. On week 4 the same friends came over and I made them smell it and they were surprised. Still, if I hadn't told them it was last month's chicken, we totally would have thought it was fine. All in all, the chicken lasted six weeks.

And also through the magic of preservatives mayonnaise no longer requires refrigeration. How do I know it's true and safe? Because my local health inspector told me so when he found my catering jug of mayo in the walk-in. Yep, health inspectors are now trained that open mayo can stay out on the counter.

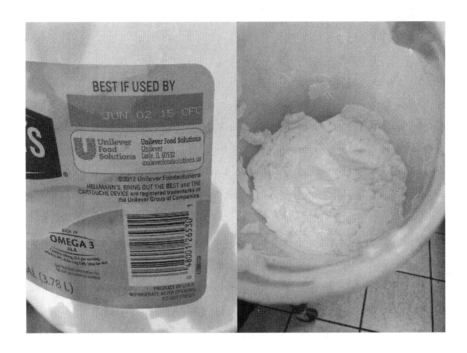

So Of course. I needed to test this theory. Here's my mayo, never put in the fridge and "expired" since June 2, 2015, but it's still looking fresh as daisy, in December 2015.

Processes:

Just watch the show The Food Factory a couple of times and you'll get the idea.

Hot liquids are put into plastic tubes, liners, bottles, and packages multiple times throughout the production process. Some plastics get baked, some get dunked in hot water to seal, some get baked, chilled and frozen so that you can then microwave them and put the through a second heating process. Products like organic gourmet baby food in pouches and Tofurkey ^{tm} get cooked or pasteurized in the plastic, twice. Plastic is great for the food industry; it's cheap! It's cheaper than glass with less breakage and loss, it's THE way to move forward for convenient one-time use. There are no labeling requirements for the chemical contents in the packaging. In fact, it is considered in the biz to be proprietary information and often patented... soo it's a secret.

But, were learning new info and terms like BPA's, PHOA's hormone disrupters, endocrine disrupters and so on and so on. So I reached out to the Consumer Reports and here's what they said:

"Ms. Eliot, unfortunately we do not have any information on proving if plastics are safe for cooking or any if anyone else has done this testing.

Please be assured that our readers' feedback plays a strong role in the work that we do. Because of this I have taken the liberty of sharing your feedback with the appropriate members of our staff for their review and future consideration.

Consumer Reports is committed to making your experience positive and informative.

Sincerely,

Celeste P.
Representative"
Customer Care

001689127B

If and how these chemicals challenge our gut linings is not known at this time. If it's on the shelf, it just means it's for sale.

While "added" preservatives are listed on the ingredient panel, preserving chemical dips and sprays are not. Now since I regularly cook for those with highly compromised gut linings and health, I started doing a little research of my own.

Shelf life tests are a great way to find out if there's a new process in play that may be challenging. If something seems different, buy one, open it, and leave it on the counter. By not refrigerating, you're speeding up the process and you'll know within 5 days or so if mold is not growing or sprouts aren't sprouting.

Our produce sources are constantly rotating inside the food matrix with different farms contributing as their fields grow or yield. And of course we have cold storage and many other preserving methods in place. When potatoes, onions, and garlic stopped sprouting, I needed to understand how this would impact my clientele, and if items not on the dirty dozen lists needed to be on mine. Garlic, onions, and potatoes are almost sacred to me. Their skins provide vitamins, nutrients, detoxing antioxidants, and they taste damn fine! And the whole onions and garlic being big on the anticancer food lists thing … this is a case where organic is sooo worth it, every time!

There's one more behind the scenes process I look for and it's called Irradiating or "cold pasteurization". It's when the food is exposed on ionizing radiation and the changes that occur prevent sprouting and ripening. In 1977 the FDA approved wheat, flour, red meat, poultry, pork, fresh shell eggs, vegetables, and spices as well as refrigerated and frozen uncooked meat, meat by-products, and certain other meat food products (whatever "other meat food products mean").

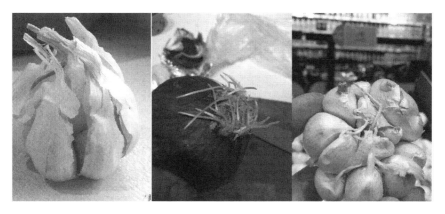

Irradiating and new tech sprays and chemical dips stop sprouting. The conventional garlic on the left never sprouted before rotting. Sprouting potatoes, onions and garlic is a very good sign that enzyme integrity is intact. To see sprouting is a good thing.

Quick Hint Shortcut: Organic cannot be irradiated. I recently reached out to Whole Foods about their policies. While we work diligently to avoid irradiated foods, we cannot guarantee that products sold in our store have not been irradiated, since many irradiated products are not required to be labeled. Customers who are looking to avoid irradiated foods should choose organic products, since United States, Canada, and European Union Organic Standards prohibit this practice.

Another process not on the label is chemical dipping for foods such as bromide and bud nip for garlic, onion, potatoes, and carrots to prevent sprouts and decay. If you want to know if these chemicals are in your food, it's very simple to know. Leave one head of garlic or one potato out on the counter for a few days. You'll know in just 7 to 10 days if your produce is not sprouting. This poor garlic never sprouted after 8 weeks.

Garlic, I see as sacred to my Italian chef soul, taste buds, and bodies of my clients. Now aside from the countless dirty old Italian men I know who personally swear by it— they say "it's the gaaalic, my fatha swore by it and I do too," as they proclaim their shtoop'n prowess being little blue pill free— garlic contains a powerful antioxidant called allicin and it repairs all sorts of cells with the benefits of controlling blood sugars and blood pressure to reducing inflammation and yeast. It's also proven to help absorption of iron and zinc.

I know, it's kitchen time, but this is something that is worth the effort

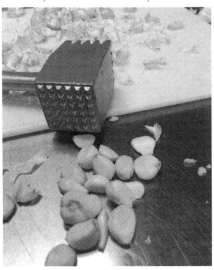

because it tastes so great, too. I'm going to show you a super quick way to peel it. Easy peasy. And warning: Once you eat delicious sautéed sweet garlic, you will be spoiled for life. Garlic just needs a little tap with a meat mallet or rolling pin, then then skin just peels off.

As for buying garlic pre-peeled, I did a few shelf life tests to see if there was going to be something "not on the label" that could impact the benefits available from the garlic.

As you can see on the label only states "fresh peeled garlic" but some how

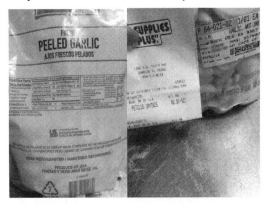

it lasts 30 day past it delivery date. In fact it didn't grow mildew or mold until late December. The garlic from China shown below also lasted a full 45 days past it sell by date.

The garlic in the plastic jug I purchased from Restaurant Depot and is a prod-

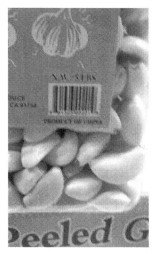

uct from China. The one in the bag is a US product distributed by US Foods, one of the largest food distributors in the country. Now let's start at the front end of this. Local mid-sized and smaller restaurants and caterers are using a "fresh" product from China. By the magic of pixie dust technology, both of these products lasted 60 days without any signs of mildew in my walk-in, plus the days it took to travel through the distribution chains from China and US.

I tried to recreate this trick. I peeled some garlic and put it a plastic container and this is what it looked like. I tried stainless steel containers too and got ten days. Stainless steel is way better! The odor is lessened and it will typically extend shelf by several days because the metal is colder than plastic.

Now I'm not sure how they create that shelf life and it's not listed anywhere on the label.

The next shelf life test I'll share for you is all about the beans. My lovely Charlotte loved her organic kidney beans as a yummy source of iron.

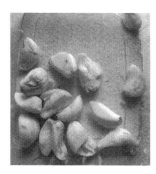

Here's what happened to organic garlic in 10 days.

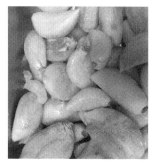

Conventional garlic after 14 days stored in stainless steel; it's clear and stinky.

But there were times when her weekly intake didn't change, but her body levels dropped. I wondered why this was happening beyond the obvious cancer obstacles. So I wanted to see if there was a brand or type of organic bean that would give us the most bang for the bite. So I did a shelf life test between the following:

• Conventional dried, 18 days and medium odor

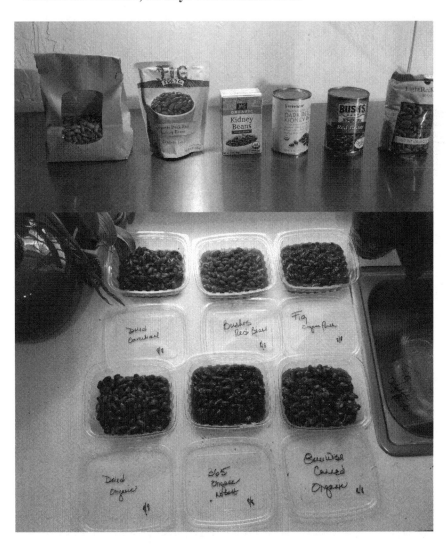

- **Organic dried, 5 days contains mildew and significant odor**
- **Bush's conventional canned, 18 days and slight odor**
- **Whole Foods 365 Organic No Salt boxed 20 days until mildew still no odor.**
- **Fig's Organic pouch, 11 days until slight odor developed**
- **Publix Green Wise Organic canned 10 days, medium odor**

Yep, the organic no salt boxed lasted the longest! I wasn't expecting that, especially without salt, since salt's one of nature's original and indigenous preservatives discovered early on.

Notice the Bush's can has a white plastic lining. This is how you know if your canned has BPA's.

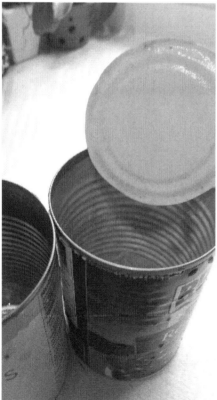

Shelf life tests are actually kind of interesting and I've learned a lot in my career. I think the most alarming thing I have learned is the lack of odor. My nose is going to be the first Italian test on the planet. We smell, we sniff, and some chefs must sniff, especially when it's bad. It's partially how we train with food. That way, if something in our kitchen smells off, we go on a safari to find it. And it's usually a stray fallen scrap that's the culprit.

Remember the saying about what company and fish have common, they both smell after two days. Now how long does the fish last? Deodorizers alarm me the most because they take away an important warning system built into the food. I wonder if our noses really can tell when something is bad or if the deodorizing technology is part of the preserving technology. It makes me wonder it's still okay to use pasta on day 20, for example, when it's made from enriched dwarf wheat flour. Yes, pasta lasts 20 days in my fridge. Yet organic pasta from Italy is moldy and sweat funky smelling by day 7.

This doesn't stink either?

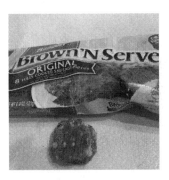

Shelf life tests are great way to test what you buy. In the next chapter, Wholesome Meal Rules will automatically steer you away from most of the disasters I just shared.

Or is it just a lie? There is a lot of misrepresented Olive Oil and honey on the market.

Here's a simple way to check your olive oil is really olive oil. Stick in the fridge. True Olive oil with congeal and thicken up as in this photo.

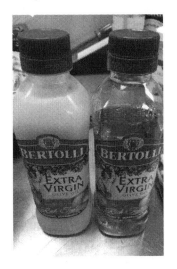

As for your honey- Buy it local and watch it drain from the hive it you can. There a huge global scandal going on right now with fake honey, sugar and corn syrup diluting true honey. Compounded with a horrible epidemic of bee hive collapse, the honey in your familiar bear plastic bottle could be fake.

CHAPTER SEVEN -THE WHOLESOME MEAL RULES

GMO is classified by the government as **"All Natural"** so the industry uses it often in their marketing. Other than that, **"All Natural"** will mean there are no artificial ingredients in the food, which is a good thing.

Enriched or fortified or vitamin-enhanced on the label means vitamin supplements have been sprinkled on top or baked in. There is a government FDA requirement that started in the 1940's that would ensure the manufacturer would restore the nutrient value of the food that their processing had stripped away. It started with cereals then crossed over to milk. Pasteurizing destroys the vitamin D, whether organic or conventional. Vitamin D should also be listed in the ingredient panel. So what kinds of supplements are added? That will vary greatly on manufacturer and the price point of the product. Most recently the cereal companies adjusted their supplement quantities because the doses were based on an adult, not a child.

Produce. Not everything needs to be organic, but the FDA tests for pesticide residues and these two groups publish the analysis. The EWG.org and consumer reports http://www.consumerreports.org/cro/health/natural-health/pesticides/index.htm and www.ewg.org Once you evaluate the price of organic, it's usually a difference of pennies. If you are going to eat the rind, peel, or skins, then I like organic, such as using the garlic skins in the bone broth.

And P.S. this list is especially helpful for dried fruits, since you typically are eating much more of the fruit, ipso facto, more of the pesticide residue.

Fats and anything that naturally contains fat needs to be the highest quality you can get your hands on. Remember how our bodies store toxins in our fats? Well so it goes for eggs, chickens, beef, dairy, butter, and plants. This is why, for example, the mercury in the fish is highest in the fattier fishes and why a New Zealand study found DDT in school cafeteria butter.

Words like organic, grass-fed, pastured (meaning the animal got sunlight), humanely raised and non-GMO are all good.

Oils I use

Coconut non-filtered and coconut-filtered. The difference is the filtered version has a less sweet coconut flavor. There is a definite coconut flavor on board. It's great for anything you want sweet, as well as Thai and Asian dishes.

Olive oil first press and just regular. First press is wonderful on salads while the regular pure olive oil is great for sauté. Organic olive oil is becoming more main stream and available now too.

Butter, organic grass fed source. Quick update: butter is back, so make it organic.

What studies show is fats increase our vegetable nutrient absorption. Clean fats are an important pairing when preparing veggie sides.

Ready for this? <u>organic grass fed butter</u> has been proven heart-healthy now because it's one of the best sources for omega-6 and omega-3 fatty acids and both are proven to reduce the risk of heart disease. These good fats also help regulate cholesterol and can help reduce high blood pressure. It's also brain food: these same omega fatty acids help create new cell membranes in the brain and support the renewal of vital brain pathways. The short-chain fatty acid Butyrate in grass fed butter has been linked to preventing neurodegenerative diseases and a proven anti-inflammatory which can prevent serious blood clots or hemorrhaging in the brain. And makes you skinny! It seems the conjugated linoleic acid in grass fed butter has been proven to reduce body fat mass especially in overweight individuals. The butyrate content helps with energy expenditure, enabling fat burn. And while Time Magazine issued a report on the benefits of butter, they just left out one thing: the fats store toxin parts.

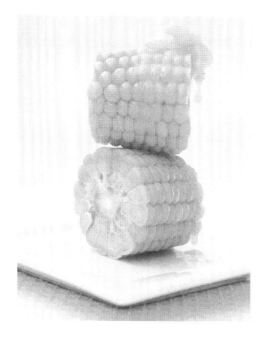

Soy, corn, canola and Palm oils must be organic. Organic canola is beginning to get some good reviews and is worth watching. Palm oil is the cheapest global oil on the market; it's rapidly deforesting Indonesia and the international food biz loves it! It's on the cardiologists' and gastroenterologists' protocols, shoved in the 'No' category because it's saturated and processed with harsh solvents.

Proteins from animals and plants naturally contain fats so the above rule applies.

Protein has essential amino acids our bodies don't make. These essential amino acids are the building blocks to creating tissue, muscle, and your skin, both inside and out. What you eat today is the skin you wear in 30 days; this is exactly a 'you are what you eat' thing.

Chicken, organic & humanely raised, is the gold standard for poultry. I'm a big fan of local and organically grown too! There are lots of farming organizations on Facebook to help you find some local chickens and eggs.

Eggs Find Local First, really. If you're buying at a grocery store, eggs should say both *Organic* and *Free Range* or *pastured* (meaning the chicken got sunlight) on the label. *Pasteurized is different from pastured. Pasteurized could mean the egg or egg product has been brought to 130 degrees for 4 minutes to kill salmonella and other issues. Or pasteurized is also the legal term used for irradiating. All those different varieties of eggs at the store are more about the marketing. Example: 'vegetarian-fed' likely means the chickens were fed GMO soy and corn.

Eggs are so important to find locally and they are easy to raise on your own. They are fresher and higher in Vitamin D. One study showed organic pastured eggs contains 1/3 less cholesterol, 1/4 less saturated fat, 2/3 more vitamin A, two times more omega-3 fatty acids, three times more vitamin E, and seven times more beta carotene than its conventional counterpart, as well as omega 3's. They taste richer and you get to support your neighbor. Win-win! You can find fresh local eggs at farmer markets and local growers on Facebook and other social media platforms. You can find these crown jewels of nutrition on Facebook. Eggs are one of those foods where it's worth the added time and effort to find them fresh. And when you do find them, stock up. A fresh unwashed and unrefrigerated egg lasts for months.

And as a chef, I know conventional eggs are more acidic. Here's the story behind that. Every seen green scrambled eggs? Well, the color has to do with the aluminum content in your pan and the acidity of the egg. Now as a badass catering chef, I learned how to get rid of that by adding a few drops of lemon juice or dollop of sour cream to the raw egg mixture before cooking. Change the PH to more neutral to stop the interaction and discoloration.

Beef: grass-fed and organic are the words you're looking for; it's level 5 at Whole Foods. This purchase is worth double points in this game. Grass-fed grazed cattle not only are on anti-cancer nutrition protocols because the meat is so nutrient-dense, but the positive sequestration of carbon from our atmosphere is huge. Follow Peter Blyck and Carbonnation on twitter.

Quinoa gets its own spot because it earned its nutrition. Quinoa is a complete protein containing all eleven amino acids.

Rice & Beans combo pack. It's the combining of these two carbs that create a complete protein. I like dried organic here because it's super cost-effective, creating an enormous land pack for pennies.

Seafood. I can no longer recommend fish as wholesome food with a few exceptions of wild Alaskan-caught seafood, clean aquaculture-farmed shrimp, and muscles. As you seek out sustainable clean sources for you, check out RDM Aquaculture in Indiana. This company is on forefront of clean shrimp technology and may know of other clean farms near you or ways to source their products.

Dairy, milk & cheese must be organic or imported. It is enriched to put the vitamin D back in, whether conventional or organic.

American conventional dairy sales have been declining since 2009 for a reason. It is a disaster and no wonder our allergies to dairy are on the rise. Dairy has been on the M & M (measure and manage list) for cancer diets, autism, and celiac disease, as well as most athlete's nutrition protocols for the past eight years that I know of. Conventional dairy is de-odorized, homogenized, pasteurized, and has flavors added. It likely contains antibiotics, which remove the beneficial probiotics and enzymes and destroy the vitamin D that was originally in the milk. And some brands still are loaded with hormones like RBST, which is banned in other countries around the world. This quart of milk smelled fresh 32 days past the sell by date. I was so surprised by this I couldn't resist taking it on to a recent appearance on the Holly Grove Radio Show.

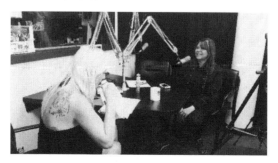

**Fun Fact: It takes 4 ounces of milk to make 1 ounce of cheese; so eating a standard 2-ounce slice of cheese is like drinking a glass of milk.

Organic fermented dairy such as cheese, sour cream, crème fraiche, and yogurt are better choices. The fermentation of raw dairy creates super beneficial probiotics for gut flora, so look for the words or seal for Live & Active Cultures. I look for imported cheeses, raw cheeses, and specialty US cheeses. Raw dairy is hot button in the food conversation. I like it for myself personally, but I do not recommend it for children or folks with compromised health. The risks if you don't know the farm are not worth the benefits. I know the farm where my raw milk comes from and it's my decision for me. In Europe it's a different food system and they are so clean you can buy raw milk from vending machines.

Wheat. Must be organic. Big changes have occurred in this industry. I don't know if it's the genetic alterations, if it's been irradiated (as approved by FDA in 1977), or its other chemicals and technology that they don't have to put on the label. The wows of wheat can be summed up thusly: the dwarf species of wheat created and fed to us in 1980's hasn't gone so well for us. Remember when flour got mealy bugs? No more. I found this bag of flour last year that expired in Dec 22 2011, so I saved it ☺. Four years later, still no bugs or breakdown whatsoever. If I didn't look at the date, I would totally use this flour.

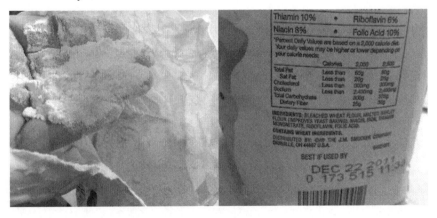

Wheat is an original food source; we used to have over two thousand different species growing, and civilizations were built on it. Pennsylvania Amish still grow food old school style and there are a lot of organic flour companies online now, and fortunately there are wonderfully crazy farmers out there starting up artisan flour businesses.

Again, let's not throw the baby out with the bath water. Let's revert back to the varieties of wheat that we can stomach.

I'm Italian and am having trouble giving up the pasta. The good news is the organic semolina from Italy is still pretty old school A big countermeasure to the carb spike is to make sure your meal is rich in fiber and that your pasta is cooked al dente. So Primavera please!

Salt needs to contain vital minerals. If not, it is just processed sodium chloride often called table salt. It's been enriched with iodine supplement and stripped of the minerals, which tends to lead to overeating and it just tastes flat. Look for labels that say it contains vital minerals. Pink Himalayan Sea Salt, Celtic sea salt, and grey sel are my favorites. Warning: once you go with vital mineral sea salts, you'll be spoiled for life by the taste. It's how I get clients off of MSG; it's that good.

MSG. Monosodium glutamate, aka hydrolyzed yeast, aka natural flavors, and aka at least twelve more legal names just to trick you. MSG is the darling of the food industry; it is an excitotoxin, a trick. Your brain thinks it tastes better than it does. And it's an appetite stimulant, too, so you eat more. MSG is a "no" on every doctor protocol I ever got. It stimulates neuron receptors. Neuron receptors allow brain cells to communicate with each other, but when they're exposed to excitotoxins, they fire impulses at such a rapid rate that they become exhausted. Glutamate is vasoactive - meaning it changes the diameter of the blood vessels – and that's one reason why the cardiologists protocols are so concerned with MSG, since it can cause blood vessels to constrict. Cancer docs don't like it either because their research equates MSG as cancer fertilizer. And yet the food biz jams it into food marketed for children. Now MSG is classified as a toxin by my state's food health service codes but it's sold in ½ gallon jugs. Go figure.

Since MSG is an excitotoxin, it also stimulates the brain centers just like heroin does, so some clients feel actual withdrawal. If MSG has been in your diet and your doctors have not instructed to you immediately remove it for health concerns, then I recommend reducing your intake weekly by mixing your favorite seasoning mix with Himalayan pink. Create a batch for your cooking and increase your salt to MSG ratio, and quickly you'll end up liking your food better without the MSG salty weird feeling in your mouth after you eat it. Also you'll quickly not have the addictive bingeing triggers kicking in.

Sugar I like organic molasses, local honey, organic honey, medicinal honeys, and organic cane sugar. Molasses and honey are the only two sugar sweeteners permitted in most cancer protocols, because they each offer some additional benefits such as calcium and B vitamins in the molasses and pollen in the honey. I like organic here, too, for lots of reasons. Honey is another sacred food for medicinal purposes. The whole beehive collapse crisis is driving a black market with international distribution and that has been traced back to bottles in US grocery stores. So if you want to know if you're really getting honey, then you want local or organic.

You do need some glucose for good health, but it's not that much. In Jan the Federal Government released the new Dietary Guidelines, recommending daily intake to be no more than 10% of daily calories. These measurements have been quantified as the following by Dr. Robert Lustwig's studies reported on by 60 minutes Sanjay Gupta's report Toxic Sugar.
http://www.cbsnews.com/video/watch/?id=7417238n

150 calories or 37.5gram or 9 teaspoons a day for men

100 calories or 25 grams or 6 teaspoons for adult woman

64 calories or 16 grams or 4 teaspoons for children over 8

48 calories or 12 grams or 3 teaspoons per day for

children 4 to 8 years' old

Translation: these amounts mean basically no sugar. Quick. Go check the sugar content of your baby food, breakfast cereal or toaster breakfast pastry. According to this new science, every morning millions of kids exceed their full day's limit of sugar before 8 a.m. You would know this if it were listed on a food label. But oddly there is no government regulation for sugar on food labels. Somehow that part's been left blank. How strange. And I say this with love in my heart. ☺ Your teaspoon from your drawer likely equals 1.5 to 2 measured teaspoons.

Studies prove anything higher increases cholesterol, inflammation, and generally challenges your gut lining, brain, and body. T'aint much, baby! Some doctors want patients to go cold turkey and some suggest a stepping down period. Since I don't have any health issues, thank God, my journey involved stepping down and cutting my intake by 50% every 5 or 10 days until I reached my 200 calorie goal. But the God's honest truth is, for obvious career influences, I am personally still wrestling with sugar to the tune of about 400 calories per day. Now please don't get deterred by this high bar or my inability to fully achieve it. I find weight loss is still possible, body repair is still available to me, and my clients are still in the process of achieving the goal. You will find your own balance and be able to do your best.

Reducing sugar reduces pain. Track that!

Here's what I need you know: It's not your fault! Sugar, MSG, and artificial flavors ALL have addictive qualities and impacts on the brain. That's why it's so freaking hard. Want to know how to crush a sugar craving? Eat fats and proteins which are conveniently put into nuts, imported cheeses, Snack Bites, and the protein pancake recipe in our plan. Emotional Freedom Tapping (EFT) is also a good diversion and gives me something else to do with my mind, other than running the scenarios of what I can do with butter, oatmeal, and honey… dude, I'm dangerous.

The Wholesome Meal Rules

Organic - Is free of GMO's and artificial chemicals.

"All Natural" - means there are no artificial ingredients in the food which is good, but it could contain GMO,'s. Check for soy, corn, canola and citric acid. If these ingredients are present look for the words non-GMO.

Enriched - fortified or vitamin-enhanced terms on the label means vitamin supplements have been sprinkled on top or baked in.

Produce - follow the www.ewg.org and www.consumerreports.org clean produce lists.

Fats - kep them real and buy the best you can afford, you're worth it! Coconut oil, Olive oil and organic butter. Soy, corn, canola and palm oils must be organic and minimally processed

Proteins - organic is best.

Eggs - local and organic is best. Organic and pastured from the store is good too. It's just not as fresh as local.

Grains - organic is best. For a few extra cents you change the world.

Seafood - I no longer recommend seafood as part of a wholesome meal.

Dairy, Milk & Cheese - must be organic or imported. Organic fermented dairy such as cheese, sour cream, crème fraiche, and yogurt are better choices. Live & Active Cultures. I look for imported cheeses, raw cheeses, and specialty US cheeses.

Wheat - must be organic.

Salt - needs to contain vital minerals. If it doesn't say contains vital minerals on the label you are missing out on 84 of them. Pink Himalayan & Celtic Sea Salts are 2 that I recommend.

Sugar - I like organic molasses, local honey, organic honey, medicinal honeys and organic cane sugar in moderate amounts.

CHAPTER EIGHT - THIS GIRL WAS ON FIRE

Over the years I continued to cook for clients with various illness and I learned. In 2005, my personal journey began when I was on fire. Yep, I caught on fire. Apparently it takes a lot to get my attention. It was a fierce Rosh Hashanah cooking accident where a propane burner with a pot of oil caught, and the next thing I knew, it was all orange, I was yelling, and I jumped into the pool. When I hopped out of the pool, I handed off cooking instructions to my other chef on-site and drove myself to the hospital, having a cig on the way. (True.) When I got to the ER, I honestly expected some burn cream and stuff, not four days of hospitalization and a surgical skin graft, where the skin was cut off my left thigh and applied to my left hand. Shock was an awesome thing for me!

After surgery I remember the nurses checked my finger tips for blood flow every few hours. Apparently there was a significant risk I could lose my hand. My single mom body, all inflamed and riddled with cortisol, 80 pounds overweight and in desperate need of healing was a mess but still strong, thank God. I entered a 3-month rehab experience that would change me forever. I am grateful I knew the right question to ask my doctors… ready for it? What nutrients is my body looking for to make skin? Because I seem to need to make some more quick. The answer given was Vitamins A, C, E, and zinc. So I Googled 'foods rich in Vitamin A', then 'foods rich in Vitamin C', etc. etc. and voila! I had my go-to meal, which was turkey, spinach, and avocado, which I prepared dozens of different ways and ate twice a day for nearly three months.

On my next follow up appointment, the Cleveland Clinic doctors got all excited when they saw my hand. While I saw something that more re sembled Frankenstein but purple with black stitches, they saw and a 98% skin adhesion rate. Apparently anything over 35% is considered a success. They asked me stay a little later and parade of doctors came by to peek and they took photos, too.

Now I wasn't the best physical therapy patient at first, and setting aside three 90 minute windows every week in October, going into catering season, was so not happening, until my therapists looked me dead in eyes and asked, "Do you want your hand back or not?" Boom. She had my attention. She went on to say there is only a brief window of opportunity for us to make that happen, and the only way is with all of this therapy. And this created the best habit ever. I was forced to set aside dedicated time for me, doctor's orders for hand therapy. Once hand therapy was over, I re-dedicated that time to the rest of me. And bite by bite, workout by workout, I have lost 80 pounds and gained physical strength and stamina I have never know before, ever. I've never before enjoyed such a strong body and ally in life. I was born plump and continued on that same physical path for most of my life. I had a couple of years of thin during my 20s, but I have never before been fit. I also quit the pack-a-day habit and the two daily shots of scotch at night to numb the pain. I thank God I caught on fire, because I do know this: I wouldn't be feeling as good as I do today, had I not learned how to heal.

Lesson: The lessons here: Ask the right questions and invest in your healing. It's the best time and money you will ever spend.

CHAPTER NINE – FOOD IS POWER

DJ and ATA

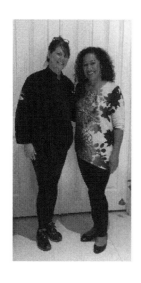

From 2008 to 2011 I served the Johnsons, and it was during this time that a unique opportunity arose. For the first time ever in my career, I was purchasing and cooking for someone very sick and someone very healthy on the very same day. And on this day I was cooking for both Ata and Dwayne Johnson and his crew. DJ is, well, a beast and his mom, Ata, was battling Stage III lung cancer, who by the way, gave cancer a fierce and massive smack down, I must say. So there I was at Whole Foods with two carts, one for Ata and one for the DJ and crew. In my mind they were totally different clients, recipes, and menus. But there I was tossing in broccoli for Ata, broccoli for DJ, chicken for Ata, chicken for DJ, spinach for Ata, no spinach for DJ— he hates spinach— grass-fed beef, sweet potato, white potato for Ata and ditto for DJ. And there I was staring at the contents of these carts and I understood— this message hit me like a rock— the right food for sexy badass muscle is also right for massive healing. It's all the same information, the same language, and the same communication of original sources of vitamins and minerals that impact the physical experience. Food is power; it's the most basic ingredient in the building blocks of our bodies.

So the lesson here is this: Food is power.

While cooking for the Johnsons, I observed one more lesson for you: they process pain differently than most. They process pain as good and as healing. Sure the injury sucked, but the rehab discomfort is good, not to be feared or avoided but embraced and used. Pain has its purpose, too.

CHAPTER TEN -TOP 6 GAME CHANGERS

As I served top pro athletes, I began to see an important pattern that created their success. Here are the top 6:

** the following info on hydration is not for folks with seizures, epilepsy, or other brain disorders. I recommend you consult with your physician for your best hydration schedule. Some studies related to the ketogenic diet show seizures decrease when the brain is slightly dehydrated. So this is delicate stuff and should be further explored to be understood as much possible to navigate the condition.

1 Hook up your hydration! I first got my real peek at what Hooking Up the Hydration looks like while delivering to various athletes' homes and such. The first time I saw a gajillion thermoses in the cupboard, I honestly thought, "Huh, that seems a little excessive." lol Look at me now. This is my daily diligence: six 16 ounce canisters of "hooked-up hydration". Some days it's just water and other days I'll pop a few slices of cucumber, lemon, a teaspoon of chia seeds, and a scoop of glutamine. It varies based on the challenges of my day.

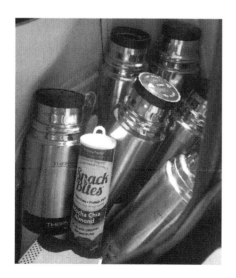

"Hydration is a huge opportunity to offer your body what it needs to thrive and it's critical to your body's performance. 60 percent of our bodies is composed of water, 75 percent in our muscles, 85 percent in our brains; it's like oil to a machine," explained Dr. Roberta Lee in a CBS report where they reported an estimated 75% of Americans are chronically dehydrated.

Trainers and Athlete's like Terry Kirby recommend water intake needs to be half your body weight in fluid ounces, minimum, for basic performance. Dr. Bret Emery recommends more when drinking anything caffeinated. Dr. Kimmi Stultz, clinical pharmacist, adds bone broth to her hydration schedule. I heard Dr. Paul Check lecture on the impact of dehydration on degenerative disc disease and I learned those spongy tissues between your bones need hydration, too. Huh, go figure: so the drinking coffee and slumping at your desk isn't the best plan?

Do you know what the first signs are if you're dehydrated? Yawning and pain. So the next time you experience either one, say cheers and chug a thermos of water. Do a self-check in five minutes and if you're feeling much better... then you know.

Signs for mild, chronic, to severe dehydration according to John Higgins, MD, associate professor of cardiovascular medicine at the University of Texas in Houston, and chief of cardiology at Lyndon B. Johnson General Hospital:

Weakness, yawning

Dry mouth

Pain , Muscle cramps

Food cravings, sweets

Dry skin

Fever and chills

Lightheadedness (especially when standing)

Headaches

Nausea and vomiting

Heart palpitations

Decreased urine output

Fun Fact: Pain management drugs typically have dehydrating effects on the body. Check your script and increase your ounces until you feel you're past the effects.

You need the water, but not the plastic. Plastic bottles, sippy cups, liners in cans and pouches, and disposable plates with shine or coating have not been proven safe. Current science is now measuring hormone disrupting chemicals such as phthalates, BPA's and PFOA's. They are also not getting recycled, as you might think.

Techknow's interview with Susan Collins, president of the non-profit Container Recycling Institute, states the recycling industry only actually "recycles" 5 to 7% of what we put in the recycle bins. And we only put an estimated 9% in the bin in the first place. While the goal is 1-1 recycling, we are soooo not there yet. In fact that means for every 180 items you buy and use that can be recycled, the industry recycles about 1; 179 other items are not.

We Americans use 38 billion bottles of water a year and it's estimated 75% of Americans function dehydrated. If you all take my advice about hydration and use plastic, your exposure to these chemicals is increased, the environment is screwed, and lastly you get ripped off.

Did you know you overpay by 2000% for water when you buy it in a bottle vs tap? Municipalities around the country are doing such a great job with tap water that the bottled water companies are using it. And even with the beverage industries costs involved in packaging and distribution, the beverage industry looks to enjoy a 90% profit margin, as profiled in HBO's special The Weight of the Nation. Sadly, even in times of severe drought, Nestle ^{tm} is refusing to reduce operation in California.

Home refrigerator and tap filtration technology has advanced just like everything else. I recently learned the city of Pompano in Florida uses reverse osmosis technology. So if you think the water in a bottle is safer or cleaner, that's only really true if you are living in a distressed area of the planet. Bottled water is a great thing for times of disaster and tainted water systems.

I like stainless thermoses because they are super easy to clean, they hold the correct temperature for about 24 hours, and they don't hang onto odors.

Now I definitely don't have the patience to stand at the fridge waiting for the water to filter out and fill up 6 thermoses, so here's a MacGyver.

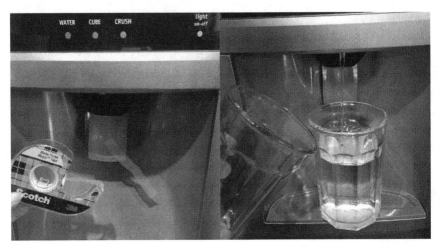

I tape the back flap down to leave the water on. Then I just need to listen for when the glass is full and quite, then switch glasses, pour into my thermos and multi task with making coffee for playing with my pussy cats; the three things that start my day.

Ed Bagley, our generation's sustainable eco-guru, likes stainless and so does Oprah with her stainless straws. I say stainless is the new green. ☺ And here's my answer to Nestle and bottled water companies that refuse to shut down operations even during times of drought.

Green juicing is an awesome player in your hydration game. I'm not saying fruit juice or sweet smoothies, I'm talking green veggie juices with ½ of your favorite fruit and whatever else you'd like to have on board. If you don't a have a juicer, get one. Put it on your holiday list, have your Facebook friend go fund it, or find a local juice bar. Juicing experts all agree: significant amounts of nutrients are lost; they oxidize inside 24 hours unless preservatives are onboard. So if you don't have a juicer at home, help you and a local business thrive; get your butt to your local juicer.

2 Dinner IS the most important meal of the day. I learned this from many of my clients and from Dr. Bret Emery at Emery Behavioral Medicine. Bret consulted for the Atlanta Braves baseball players, professional golfers, members of Lance Armstrong's U.S. Cycling Team, the Florida Panthers hockey team, and little old me. I owe my first shifts towards success to him. He told me "once my clients get their dinner on track, everything else falls into place." He referred several clients to me over the years and he was right. And here's why:

It's when we sleep that our bodies repair and restore. Cooking for athletes, I learned their training schedule often looked like this: wake up ridiculously early, get in a pre-workout mini meal of protein & carbs, work out like beast, get in protein and carbs. Go home, get in more protein and carbs, and then sleep. You see, the growth hormone is only released during sleep and those few seconds of massive intense physical challenge, like those screamers when you're lifting weights. Growth hormone is the messenger for "fix" and "fix" goes everywhere, not just to the quad you just shredded, but to your lung tissue, intestinal tissue… "fix" goes everywhere. So loading up on nutrients right before the time your body needs them most to "fix" tends to get outstanding results. And when you restore well, you wake up refreshed. So if you're not waking up refreshed, get your dinner on track and see if that helps you as much as it has all of my clients. So that means

1 (bioavailable nutrition) + 1 (restorative sleep cycle) = Thrive!

You should quickly feel much better from these first two daily disciplines; I often evaluate what I want to have for dinner based on how my next day is shaping up. If I can chill or sleep in, then I may splurge; but if I have a big day where I need to be on my game, then I eat like it.

Now I know you thought breakfast was the most important meal of the day. That's actually more marketing than science. Quick! Three guesses and the first two don't count. Guess whose health magazine first coined the phrase, "Breakfast is the most important meal of the day"? Come on... here's a hint: his last name starts with the very "special" letter "K". Yep. Dr. John Harvey Kellogg in 1917. The facts are: he was a doctor, a cereal manufacturer, and the editor of Good Health, the self-proclaimed "oldest health magazine in the world" at the time. To be fair, he was promoting an easily absorbable meal for around 300 to 500 calories to folks in 1917, a time when the majority of us woke up lean and healthy, ready to perform a day of physical hard labor— something many of us could not do today. For some of us, weight and health challenges can be so severe, folks can barely put their clothes on in the morning; this is for real, no joke. Perhaps it is time for an update on this message? Oh hang on, my smartphone just got a tweet from Dr. Mercola on a new study about the benefits of intermittent fasting for folks like me looking for ways to #createthespaceforsuccess #inducehealing and #yourbodyissmarterthanyourhonorollkid. So while 4 out of 5 nutritionists agree that eating a donut is better than skipping breakfast, folks reading the newer science favor skipping if you don't feel hungry as long as you are not a diabetic or on any blood sugar regulating meds. The bottom line is there are a lot of published studies on both side of the fence, and depending upon what condition you are in, your health will dictate if breakfast is part of your solution or part of your problem in the current moment. You should wake up hungry and in search of protein, but if your gut lining is torn up from last night's dinner, it may be good idea to give your system a chance to autocorrect.

3 Pay Attention to how you feel. Athletes and sick people more than anybody else I know, pay attention to how they feel. These four words, how do you feel, are so important they are ALWAYS the first thing out of the doctor's mouth, right? It's because when you're feeling better, you're healing better. That's why after every meal I ask my clients to log how they feel, physically and emotionally. This offers the big clues to help you identify the foods that challenge you and find your power foods to thrive.

Check in with yourself 30 minutes after you eat. Are you feeling strong and good or are you exhausted, bloated, dehydrated, congested, struggling, or aggravated? Quick clue: if you sneeze during or after your meal, there's an awfully good chance you are having an allergic response. I was on a phone consult the other day when my client began clearing her throat repeatedly. I asked how long she'd been dealing with the tickle in her throat. She actually hadn't noticed she was even doing it, and she then told me she was eating a yogurt. And while she wasn't aware she was allergic, she was clearly having a reaction. She loves her yogurt, so I recommended she shift to organic to at least determine if it's a true dairy allergy or an allergy to the "all that jazz" in it that triggered her immune response. There's a lot of autoimmune stuff going on with this client, so obvious triggers like congestion are quick clues. Remember: even organic foods can challenge you if you are allergic.

4 M & M; measure and manage, don't judge it, evaluate it. As you initially focus your nutrition and health, you'll want to fully understand and embrace your areas in need of improvement. As Terry Kirby is fond of saying, "The quicker you know your weakness, the quicker you can do something about it. Chase your weakness." Instead of gorging your excuses with judgment words like 'bad', 'never', and 'avoid', just recognize it, measure it, and then take action to manage it. Success had two moving parts. Just like in football, you want to remove the obstacles and push forward. My workout chats with Terry Kirby also helped me see this one. Do you see obstacles to your success? What are they? And how do you remove them?

What are the daily diligences that move you forward?

5 Eat something raw and organic with every meal. Claire Marino was the first client to instill this in my repertoire. Later, my research of enzyme-deficient foods fully grounded this. While no grocery store can guarantee their foods are not irradiated unless the product is organic, you can increase your digestive enzyme by eating something raw and organic at every meal.

I had the pleasure of cooking the family meal for most nights for Dan Marino and Family from 2002 to 2004. All the kids were home when I started there and family meals were often filled with friends, family, and love. Every time I think of the importance of eating something raw every day, I think of Dan and Claire. Every night Claire made sure there was a great big salad for everyone and a fruit platter. Dan would also ask me to think of more creative ways to make his salad. Getting creative with macerating fruits and marinated veggies I learned here. My go to is a bite or two of fermented cabbage; that way I get the added dose of probiotics with digestive enzymes for more bang in my bite.

On a side note, it's here where I learned how to speak with love to my child. This was not something I learned in my home as child, so when I overheard bits and pieces of the family conversations, I soaked it in like sponge. No matter what got thrown out at the evening dinner table, I could hear Claire's loving and firm voice gently guiding the conversation and keeping it productive at every turn. I credit Clair and the lessons I overheard for the closeness I have with my own daughter and I am forever grateful.

Top 6 Game Changers
for Success

• Hook up your hydration!

• Dinner IS the most important meal
of the day

• Pay Attention

• M & M - Measure and manage
don't judge it, evaluate it

• Eat something raw and organic
with every meal

• If health permits, you must have a
splurge meal at least once a week.

CHAPTER ELEVEN –WHEN FOOD AND MEDICINE WORK IN HARMONY

So fast forward almost twenty years from my experience cooking for Dr. Burton to when my phone rings and I hear the most urgent nutrition dynamic I ever was asked to cook. David inhaled a brain-eating, antibiotic-resistant bacteria while traveling in Europe. While I'm not privy to all the details, several operations were involved and he was placed on <u>the only</u> antibiotic available and it only worked if his sugars didn't go above 130. David is a Type 2 Diabetic who for the past 35 years managed his condition with meds and not his diet. So on a good day, his sugars hovered in the 150s.

Now I fully understood the gravity of what I was asked to cook and I knew I had this! For David I cooked what I always cook: beans from scratch, organic meats, lots of interesting veggie sides, interesting carbs deliciously seasoned, and poached fruits. I also brought nuts to peel or shell, to Atack his night munching game. When I dropped off his food, I did a quick sort of naughty and nice rundown of his fridge and shared what I knew about "how not to" jack up his sugars with artificial sugars and chemicals. And finally we reviewed his portion sizes and how to quickly heat up his meals.

I heard nothing for days and days, which usually means good news. On Day 6 I called. I gently asked, "How's it going?" David's Type 2 diabetes medication was reduced and re-dosed three times in the first week alone because the diet was working so well, even with everything else going on in David's body chemistry; his body still fully recognized and used the nutrient-dense foods to reset and heal. That's how it works, folks. Think of your food as "Safe Base". It's the place the doctors send their patients to heal. Clean, targeted nutrition using wholesome ingredients has no downside, no risk, no recalls.

Lesson: You can always rest in safely in the intelligence of nature's whole foods.

Now when I say safe, those words mean something quite different when it comes to food labeling; the words 'safe' and 'nutritious' are a lot like cognac and brandy. Not all "safe" foods are nutritious but nutrition foods are indeed safe by definition. So watch for the food manufactures getting recalled and ask why? So, for example, eggs and salmonella. Why we are even accepting this and buying conventional, pasteurized, irradiated or liquid eggs? If the way they produce is so dirty, as in every hen is contaminated with salmonella, they are doing something wrong. The next answer is to not add processes to fix it, like pasteurizing, irradiating, or serving when fully cooked. The last answer is to fix the filthy conditions that created it in the first place. Somehow European countries, Asia, and even third-world countries provide nutritious eggs and raw dairy. I know we can, too. We just need to ask for it and by that I mean *Buy* That.

CHAPTER TWELVE - HOW TO CREATE YOUR FOODS SCRIPT

***Before you upgrade your food, talk to your doctor; especially if you're taking any medications. Here's the deal: if you are on medication that works along with diet and exercise, and you have not correctly put those two pieces into your game, then you are in for such a big surprise; let me tell you.

Your conversations should include how any and all medications you are taking will be effected by weight loss, increased hydration, and sweating. For example, every time— and I mean every time— a client with Type 2 diabetes loses the first 15 to 30 lbs., they one day suffer a hypoglycemic episode because the med dose is too high and it's dropping their sugars too far. It involves shaking and sweating and it's alarming. So understanding what this feels like to step down off your medications and having a game plan on what to expect is very helpful. Health dynamic shifts so getting a current read on what's going on is very helpful too.

I always say, 'Don't eat what your neighbor eats, don't eat what your trainer eats, and definitely don't eat what Larry the Cable Guy eats.' You need to eat what you need. We are all in our own space in the spectrum of the health dynamic. We all have our own combinations of impacts going on and properly recognizing where you are right and what you need to heal is the quest. I call this process 'creating your own Foods Script'. Some athletes only eat one or two veggies, but you better be darn sure they are the nutrient-dense ones.

I like to create my foods lists in excel. So I have a nice column and a naughty column. At the end of this process you want to focus your purchases on the foods that are part of your solution. To create your foods script, do a little research on foods that benefit your specific health dynamic. Here are some search examples for you. Remember to include your pain and fatigue.

Foods to avoid for (____Name your health condition, name your medication____) you fill in the blank.

beneficial foods for (Name your health condition or symptoms, state your age, your race, your goals)

Food and (_____medication name____) conflicts
(medication name) and hydration

These are basic examples of searches, so get creative with your searches; remember to ask the right question ;-) Then, be a good journalist; confirm it three times. Can you get three legit sources of info to confirm? To evaluate legitimacy, look for who has paid for the study. Ask if the food manufacturers need to pay for their endorsement? And view the "sources" other dietary recommendations. If you find food from the 1950's, gelatin, soda crackers, cereal, artificial sugars; then you have a sense of their education and experience.

My go-to resources are:

Dr. Axe, Dr. Mercola and Dr. Mark Hyman
Eat this and live by Dr. Don Colbert, MD
Gillian McKeith's Food Bible, how to use food to cure what ails you.

*****Note all allergies trump beneficial category, so if you are allergic, it's off your list for now. The severity of the allergy and how well you reconstruct your gut lining will dictate if you can reintroduce a beneficial food*

Cravings count. Are you experiencing any "real" food cravings? Sugar cravings and foods that have MSG triggers for you are lies. Reducing sugar reduces pain. Track that. Feeling better is a huge motivator for getting past the crazy cravings. For real cravings I mean, you're thinking; cucumbers, oranges or a thick rare steak. These are very helpful clues. Then Google, "nutrients in steak" and nutrients in cucumber, orange, etc. Look for common threads if you tracking a health dynamic. Indulge in your true food cravings, your body IS that obvious.

Creating the Daily Diligence
My most successful clients have what I call 'the daily diligence'. Every day they commit to "getting them in" the basics of their day. My daily diligence is 1 hot green tea, 1 organic apple, 6 waters, and 2 cups spinach first thing in the a.m. I take Omegas in the a.m. and in the p.m. So once you have your list of beneficial foods, let's identify the ones that will give you the biggest bang for your buck. Brainstorm ways to "get them in".

Calories count! But not for the first 5 to 10 days or 1 to 2 gut linings. I don't suggest calorie restriction for your foods script. There's a darn good chance you are nutrient deficient. Your weight is your weight and between losing 4 lbs. in 2 weeks vs reloading and resetting some of your primary systems, I'm going with restoring nutrients before calorie restriction. It's also a great time to generally learn the calorie and composition of the foods you need.

Calories Composition 101 The Basics
***Here's the short cut: Count carbohydrates first. Clients healing or working out were able to process a few extra bites of protein or fats more so than extra carbohydrates. Tracking the carbohydrates is the game changer.

Calorie compositions are from protein, fats, and carbohydrates. A basic 300 to 350 calorie meal breakdown with a 40-30-30 balance— meaning 40% of your calories are coming from protein, 30% from carbohydrates, and 30% from fat— **looks like this:**

5 ounces of protein

¾ of a cup of carbs

Unlimited veggies. (Veggies are free, but the fats or carbohydrates you used preparing them do count.)

Everything prepared with 1 tablespoon of oil max.

*** *Amounts of protein, fats, and carbohydrates may be different for you if you suffer from any conditions that limit your ability to process proteins, fats, or carbohydrates.*

A consensus of yeses puts daily calories for women at 1,200 calories and 1,500 for men for weight loss goals. By targeting the 300 calorie meal, you can eat 3 - 5 times in the day. Don't forget to account for calories from beverages and snacks.

Once you create your first calorie-targeted meal, don't just count your blessings; count your bites. Count how many bites of protein and how many bites of carbohydrates. It will give you a really good frame of reference for times when you're eating out. Be mindful of fats, sugars, and preservatives.

Now if you want more than 300 calories in your meal, then increase carbohydrates, protein, and fats accordingly, keeping a 40-30-30 balance. And that basically works out to 3 more bites of protein, 4 bites of carbs. Good fats and proteins are the keys to giving the body extra calories. There is where nuts and nut butters really can play a great role.

Cancer Nutrition is a quickly developing area of study and knowledge. Here's what I've learned thus far:

Your body goes into upside-down land. Foods you instinctively turn to that are rich in antioxidants, such as fresh produce, are wrong for most types of cancer, especially tumors. Antioxidants feed the cancer faster than your repair.

Sugar feeds cancer.

MSG feeds cancer.

Raw veggies can trigger a bacterial imbalance in the gut lining called C-diff and it is life threatening. During the most intense times in Chemo therapy folks gut linings can become super fragile. During these times steaming veggies, fruits and salads avoid this disaster. In my chapter 'Cooking Is Love', I will show you a quick and easy steam trick for salads and fruits.

Proteins and fat are the two focused sources of nutrition. This is when I first thought up and made Snack Bites. I was looking for way to get protein and fat into my client and organic nut butters and proteins I could trust were my two top missions. Combine organic nut butters and proteins for a great nutritional team. Folks taste buds are wierded out when they are going through chemo and or radiation. Sweet stuff can be repulsive, bland flavors can feel metallic, so keeping the recipe simple at first is best.

CHAPTER THIRTEEN - MEAL PLAN AND GROCERY LIST

So now you have your beneficial list of foods. Great! Next, let's make our meal plan and grocery list. Don't worry quite so much about specific recipes; instead buy the right amounts of protein, carbohydrates, veggies, fats, and flavors, then riff! Trust me. Easy peasy.

So the way I figure out the shopping is this…

First I decide how many meals I need to create.

- **Protein.** I want 4-5 ounces of protein per serving and there are 16ounces in a pound so , 1lb of protein ='s about 3 portions per pound for all cuts except ground. Ground yields 4 portions per pound. It's just food, not algebra. lol

- Going veganore; this is where I combine half of my animal protein portion with a complete vegetarian protein from either quinoa or rice and beans, which saves $$$ without sacrificing the benefits of a complete protein.

- *Vegans increase beans, quinoa and nuts

- Veggies, 1 cup or more of veggies per meal

- Fruits 2 servings per day, include fruits in your green juices

- Carbs, 1/2 to 3/4 cup portion per meal

- Fats for cooking, 1 tablespoon per meal

- Flavors, fresh herbs, extra peppers to roast, ginger or turmeric root, citrus zest, gourmet salts

Let's say I want 3 meals a day for 6 days so I'll target 18 meals.

General Grocery list for 18 meals

But you don't want 18 meals? That's okay, just calculate and reset to your needs you now know what amounts are of your wholesome meal.

Protein: $30 to $50.00

1 dozen pastured organic eggs – 6 breakfasts (or even breakfast for dinner): $8.00

4 pounds of protein or 2 pounds for veganores: $20.00 to $40.00 *vegans increase beans, quinoa and nuts

18 cups of veggies: $40.00

1 large box of spinach = 6 cups, add to protein drink or add to lunch & dinner meals- get it in!

1 head of cabbage, fermented – unlimited eating opportunity

6 cups of assorted veggies

or

1 box organic spinach plus

12 cups of assorted veggies if not making fermented cabbage

Fruit: $10.00

6 cups, or so of fruit

Organic apples for apple sauce

Carbs: $20.00

Pick 4 carbs – 4 servings each item, approx. You'll gain those 2 servings when you buy beans or quinoa, so don't worry.

Potatoes to bake, white and sweet

Beans – Yes you can make them without presoaking overnight!
*Can freeze excess

1 lb. of dried organic beans (can freeze once cooked, be prepped for next week time. Saving tip: you can freeze and increase your batch to 2 pounds if you like.)

Grains or pasta… Yes, I said pasta. Maybe it's the Italian in me, or the fact it's an ancient food, but it's not just me; most folks would like to keep a little pasta in their plan. So if that's you, too, I recommend the organic, made in Italy, and imported kinds of pasta. Cheap pasta is made with cheap flour.

In a recent shelf life test, a pan of leftover pasta from catering took 28 days to show signs of turning bad. But my organic stuff is done in 6 or 7 days, tops!

2 things you can do to make the sugars and carbs from pasta and grains less impactful:

*Cook it al dente, a recent glycemic index test showed pasta cooked al dente registered lower on the index? That's a good thing.

*Did you know: by adding more fiber into your meal, it reduces your insulin response? So make sure you eat extra veggies.

Flavors and Fats $30.00

For flavor, I really like all fresh herbs, ginger, garlic, spicy spices and tricked out salts.

Fats. You'll be using approx. 1 cup of oil for your week. Here's what you'll have. (I have them listed in priority in case you need to purchase them one at a time):

Oils - Extra virgin olive oil for low or no temp

Organic butter

Organic canola or macadamia nut oil for high temperatures

Coconut oil

Nuts - Budget $10.00 a week on nuts and seeds, great for snacking

Cheese - If you love a great imported Parmesan Reggiano and it helps you get the broccoli or spinach down, go for it!

Average price is $7.22 to $8.33 per meal   ***Ding Ding Ding, Yes, you can eat clean for the price of a drive through!!!!

***Time saving shopping tip: Pack your cold stuff together; that way, when you get home, you can shove the bags in the fridge until you're ready to cook. So keep all protein together, keep produce that requires refrigeration together and keep all other items out on the counter until ready together.

Wholesome Meal Plan #1, prep time 2.5 hours

For our purposes in this next chapter, I have developed your first meal plan. Please alter to suit your taste and amount needs. You'll quickly see where you can plug in the foods you love the way you love them cooked.

Protein Pancakes - This recipe saves me for breakfast on the run; clients love'm, grown-up and kids alike; and they are perfect for when I'm craving carbs and just want to shove a hot sweet pancake in my mouth.

Whole chicken – chicken bone broth, aka Jewish penicillin

Marinated Chicken or beef

Ground Meat options, balls, loaf, burgers

Quinoa

Baked sweet potatoes/Baked White Potatoes

Beans

Pasta

Wilted Spinach

Steamed Broccoli

Roasted veggie, steamed veggies, grilled veggies

Salad dressing   101

Salsa 101

Mayo 101

Apple sauce, fruit sauce and baby food 101

Compound organic butter

Marinara – Mama Antonello's recipe

*protein drink

Grocery List For Wholesome Meal Plan #1

1 dozen Eggs = 6 meals, protein pancakes or eggs, frittata or hard-boiled

1 whole chicken = 6 meals

1 lb. ground beef or turkey = 4 meals

1/2 lb. of steak or chicken to marinate = 2 meals

Carbs -

You need to work out your portions and what I call the "how manys"; how many portions and your choices

Oatmeal   if making pancakes, need oat flour, want granola or just love hot oatmeal

Potatoes to bake white and sweet

1 lb Beans – Yes you can make them with-out presoaking overnight! *You can freeze your extra portions and use next week.

Pasta

Veggies –

1 cup raw spinach (2 servings) in protein drink daily) 6 servings, 1 large box of spinach you buy and more.

1 head of cabbage – fermenting- unlimited eating opportunity

6 "cups", so eye it! It's okay if you buy a little more. You can roast them, steam them, grill them or sauté them.

Pick a great variety and onions and garlic count as a veggie, plus 2 large onions and 2 whole gloves of garlic for sauce

plus, your something raw and organic at every meal,

Flavors and Fats

4 cans of whole plum tomatoes with basil, imported from Italy or organic

Dried basil

Oils Extra virgin olive oil for low or no temp *need 1 cup for sauce.

Organic butter

Nuts Budget $10.00 a week on nuts and seeds, great for snacking

Cheese If you love a great imported Parmesan Reggiano and it helps you get in the broccoli or spinach down, go for it!

Fresh herbs

Ginger

Citrus for zest and juice

***Time saving tip. Pack your cold stuff together that way when you get home you can shove the bags in the fridge until you're ready to cook. So keep all protein together, keep produce that requires refrigeration together and keep items that can stay on the counter until ready together.

CHAPTER FOURTEEN - COOKING IS LOVE

Hey, quick question? Do you have to cook healthy? Or do you get to cook healthy? Think about for a second.

When you feed someone something you have invested your time, your physical attention, and creative talent into, it's love. When you cook, it's an act of love, not a chore. Have you been taught that everyone's favorite thing to make for dinner is reservations? Well then, it's time to rethink everything. It's no mystery to me why Claire Marino became an awesome cook. Dan's nummy noises alone are a game changer, but add your six children's loving nummy noises too... forget about it! It's love and the divine in the doing.

Here's the finish line, your Wholesome Meal, hot and ready to eat in 4 minutes with no microwave required. When you are prepped for success, you have your carbs, veggies, proteins, fats, and flavors ready to go.

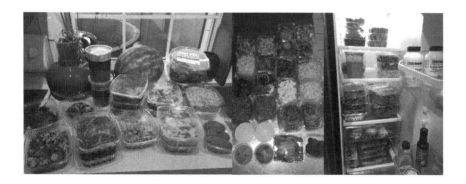

This is what a typical week in my fridge looks like. Boxes of carbs, proteins, veggies.

All you need to warm it up in 4 minutes is your Jiffy Pan and Lid Combo Trick. Okay, close your eyes, open them back up...poof! Now I'll bet you'll find one in your cabinet. Look for a small sauté pan or crepe pan and find a lid that fits. It doesn't have to match, just cover. It can even be too big. I store my Jiffy Pan in my microwave, LOL.

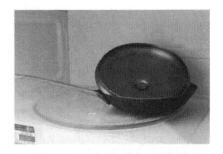

Add 2 tablespoons of water, place on high, and when the water simmers,

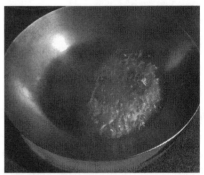

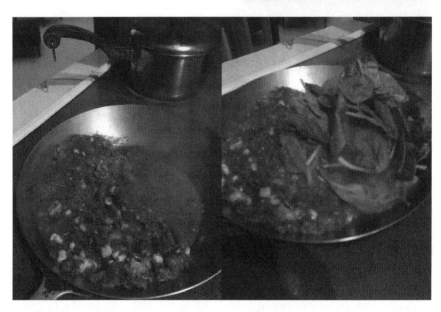

quickly add your protein, carb, veggie, and flavor base.

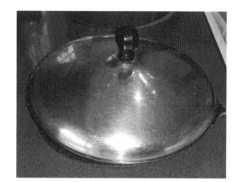

Place lid back on.

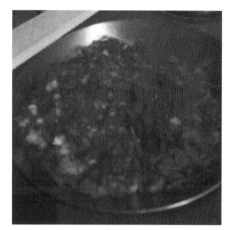

Continue to cook on high for 1 minute, reduce to low for 3 minutes, and voila, your Wholesome Meal in a jiff!

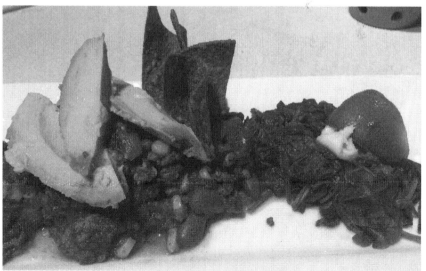

Why no microwaves?? Well, for a couple of reasons. Guys still instinctively cup their "package" if they are near one that's on.

Studies show the microwave destroys antioxidants in your food; microwaves also reconstruct protein molecules in weird ways that don't happen in conventional cooking processes which makes the meat rubbery. Crusts come out soggy, it usually cooks unevenly, food is covered in plastic, and there's a pretty high risk of a steam burn when opening it up....

Other than that, there's this....

I bought two Mexican petunias. One was fed microwaved and cooled tap water, the other fed tap water.

The plant fed microwaved water bloomed at a much reduced rate by day 3 and failed to thrive within 10 days with thinning leaves.

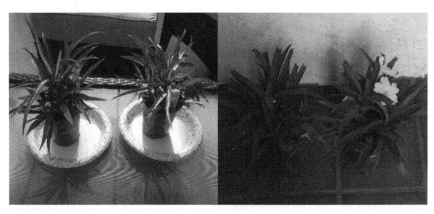

Day 1   Day 5

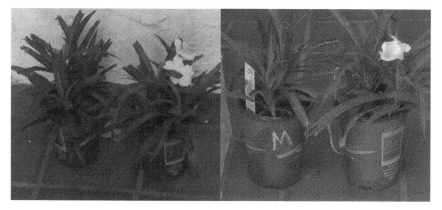

Day 7   Day 10

And finally there is this…

I recently reached out the Consumer Reports group seeking test results on plastic safety and cooking. This is something they have not tested nor could they suggest any studies proving safety. And in my research, I found the science begs for so much more.

CHAPTER FIFTEEN- KITCHEN RESET

Getting comfortable with your kitchen and equipment is key. Is your kitchen designed for delicious deeds or for your demise? I see clients climbing into drawers and cabinets, digging for sheet pans from places Cirque du Soleil performers would need a minute to think about.

Take a few minutes to quickly reset your kitchen game to make it work for you. Place the items you'll be using frequently in the cabinets closest to you and easiest for you to reach. Empty a cabinet or two that is super easy for you to access, one close to the sink counter area. It's great if it's a space that is waist-level or above for all of the equipment you will actually be using. How you place your equipment is more about how easy it to reach it versus 'oh it's flat so it should go here'.

Separate your naughty and nice spices and sauces you choose to keep. I keep a little MSG in the house and use it occasionally; but by having them separated, it just keeps me more mindful as to when I use it. When you are cleaning out the fridge, here's a shortcut: just look for sodium benzoate and citric acid. DON'T throw way the glass bottles and jars. Clean them and reuse them for your wholesome flavors and sauces.

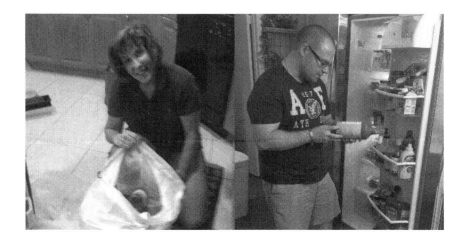

So let's assess your kitchen space, or the playing field, if you will. Do you have vases chatkey's on your stove? Is every inch of counter space in use? Clear'm off. You'll need work space and not clutter.

You will need space for storing mise while prepping and cooling food.

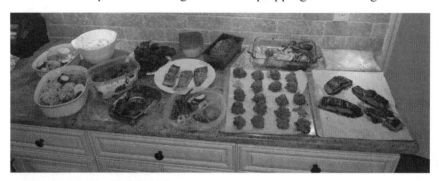

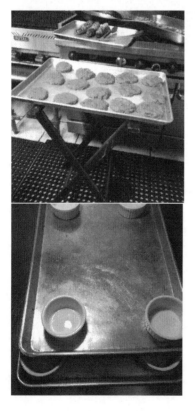

If you are counter spatially challenged, here are my two favorite MacGyvers:

The first trick involves a tray and tray jack. This baby can be set anywhere I need it! It's light weight and folds flat for easy storage.

My next trick uses sheet pans and mini-ramekins. You can use anything between the shelves to create different heights. I like the ramekins for any-time I bake kale chips and need to create more shelves in my oven.

How many steps do you have to take to throw out trash? If it's more than one, you need to move your trash can closer.

Are you right-handed or left-handed? I'm right handed so trash/scraps scrape to the right, cleaned product is placed to the left. Lefties, set the opposite direction.

Embrace washing dishes. Handwashing during your cooking session will save you so much effort and time. It takes maybe five seconds to wash out a bowl and reuse it. In fact, look for ways to use and reuse every piece of equipment you have out. The secret is in your sequencing so you can be frugal with your cleaning time. Ask yourself: is it quicker to clean it now and use it again or wait? I'm not a fan of cleaning, either for myself or my staff. I try to minimize the time we spend in total cleaning by always working clean.

I have one quick thing to say about dishwashers, hot liquids, and plastics crossing over. Sorry.... Okay, I'm done and I'll never bring it up again.

Commit to getting good with your knives. Knife 101

Your knife must be sharp. This knife sharpener sells for $6. Even the most expensive set of knives is worthless if it's dull. Good knives require a lot of time to maintain. Chefs can spend 30 minutes each night honing their blades. Me, I buy cheap knives and a sharpener.

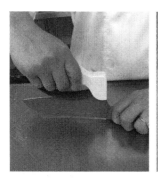 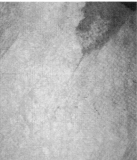

If you're holding the knife correctly, you shouldn't need to see it. You should just feel it. The trick is the blade stays on your knuckle and your fingers all remain behind the edge. It took several cases of mushrooms for me to get this. I suggest making sautéed mushroom soup or vegan burgers.

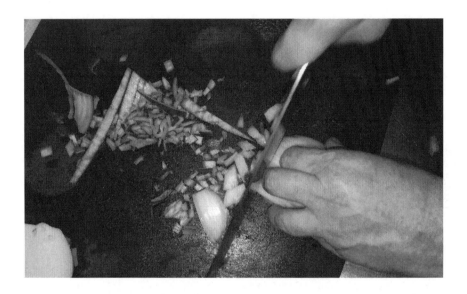

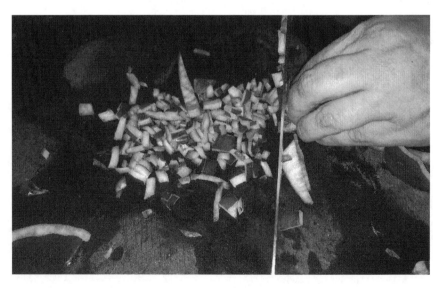

CHAPTER SIXTEEN -HELPFUL EQUIPMENT

Everything I am using is easily available online or where I purchased it, which is Restaurant Depot.

Fun Fact You don't need to have a food biz to shop there, just a business with a sales tax number. So #entrepreneur, you can shop there, too! If you don't have your own business, then find a friend who does and I'm sure he or she will take you shopping.*

What I use most every time:

Baking paper or sheet pan liners

2 large sauté pans

Braising pot for bone broth, marinara

2 small sauté pans with lids

2 medium sized mixing bowls

2 Cutting boards— I like wood best and compressed wood. One for raw meat, the other for veggies.

1 sharp 7-inch Chef's Knife

1 large meat mallet

Sheet pans – 6 to start.

Baking Pans *MacGyver foil pans

Sheet Pan Liners *saves big time on clean-up and helps you move your ingredients around

Whisk

A couple of stainless spatulas and a couple of wooden spoons to stir.

Chinoises (this is a super fine mesh strainer) Strainer with cheese cloth will do, too.

Strainer

Mandolin

Microblade which is a fine zester.

Steamer basket or metal rack that fits inside your largest pot *Mac-Gyver. You are simply keeping your food above boiling water. Easy peasy!

Meat thermometer

Containers to pack. I like using pieces that are about 24 ounces. Stainless, with or without lids, are great but can be an investment. To start – reuse any glass jars you have to empty after cleansing the fridge of products with preservatives, and even plastic zip seal bags will do to start.

Equipment to avoid

Plastic equipment. The problem with plastics, aside from the hot liquid or pan thing, is they hold bacteria— more so than wood, stainless, and glass.

Teflon and non-stick pans are getting questioned again for safety. Now it seems they release hormone disrupting chemicals calls PFOAS. Here's why I don't use them ever: One day I was going to a new client's home to cook and she repeatedly asked me about the equipment I was bringing. Since she already had a set of pots and pans, I told her I would be using hers. Easy. I arrived to the most beautiful home with bird cages and wonderful chirping sounds. We said our hellos and she inspected my boxes and baskets and bags. And finally she said, "Ok, good. I'm checking because you can't use Teflon in my house. It releases a gas that that could kill my birds." Talk about a canary in coal mine.

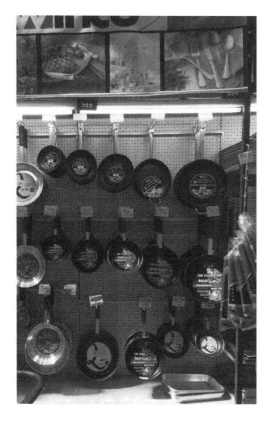

FYI, the restaurant biz and food industry haven't embraced this new science. They still very much use non-stick and sell non-stick cookware. If you are hormone challenged, avoiding non- stick coating and new tech can be another impactful step to recreating your own well -being.

CHAPTER SEVENTEEN -
THE WHOLESOME MEAL GAME PLAN

I remember the first time I did a private chef gig for 7 dinners, 2 servings each. It took me from 7:30am to 9pm at night. I swore to myself that would never, ever, never happen again. And it didn't! Over the years I fine-tuned my Game to keep it streamlined, tight, and interesting. Whether you are new to cooking or pretty comfortable in your kitchen, I hope you find this approach easy, smart, and helpful.

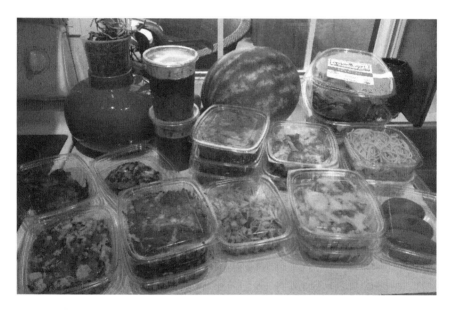

What are the two most important forces a cook controls?
Time and temperature.

To illustrate this concept, let's look at dehydrating. It's a process by which water and moisture leave the food, herbs, tomatoes, fruit, etc. And this process can happen by leaving your food uncovered in the fridge or in the oven at 125 degrees. The only difference is how long the dehydrating process will take. Both are safe at temperatures that inhibit bacterial growth.

Here's a quick reminder of our menu:

Wholesome Meal Recipes
Protein Pancakes, this recipe saves me for breakfast on the run, clients love'm grown-up and kids alike, and they are perfect for when I'm craving carbs and just want to shove a hot sweet pancake in my mouth.

Whole chicken – chicken bone broth, Jewish penicillin

Marinated Chicken or beef

Ground Meat options, balls, loaf, burgers

Quinoa

Baked sweet potatoes/Baked White Potatoes

Beans

Pasta

Wilted Spinach

Steamed Broccoli

Roasted veggies, steamed veggies, grilled veggies

Chopped Veggies, fermented cabbage, salads and salsas 101

Fats and Flavors

Salad dressing 101

Mayo 101

Apple sauce, fruit sauce 101

Compound organic butter

Marinara – Mama Antonello's recipe

*protein drink

GAME PLAN 2.5 HOUR COOK TIME

The game plan is your step by step guide to use along with your recipes so keep it handy.

If you're ADHD like me your gonna love this!!!!!

Note: you are chopping everything you intend to eat raw first.

Look for opportunities to streamline your tasks.

Use, wash, and reuse as much equipment as possible. Let your equipment availability dictate your sequencing. If you want to use two pots to cook six things, then each time a pot and burner is available it's an opportunity.

I like to shop and cook the same day. If you don't have the time or energy to accomplish both, then resist the urge to unpack your bags, just shove'm in the fridge and grab them when it's time to cook.

1. Get clean. Start your cleaning system, pull out soaps and cleansers. Get out your cutting board and knife chopping space. Get your towels handy and have a counter space flow.

2. Unpack. Sort proteins, carbs, veggies, fats, and flavors. Shove the proteins in the fridge and leave the rest out to work.

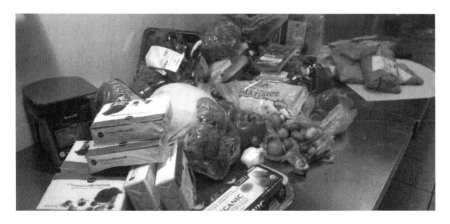

3. Washing produce – in bowl or pot – use what you have ;-) ;-)

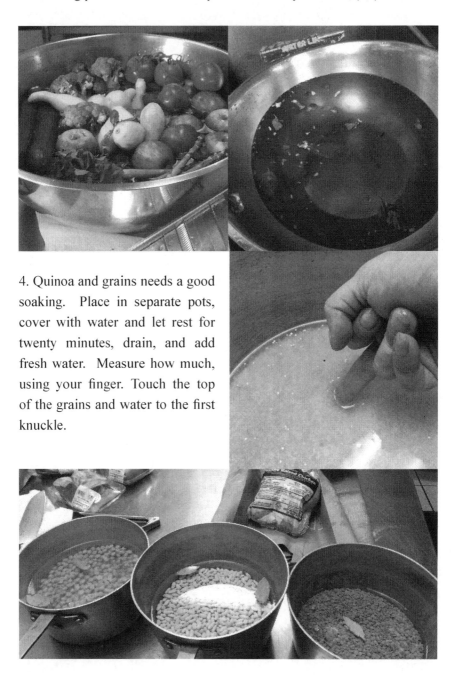

4. Quinoa and grains needs a good soaking. Place in separate pots, cover with water and let rest for twenty minutes, drain, and add fresh water. Measure how much, using your finger. Touch the top of the grains and water to the first knuckle.

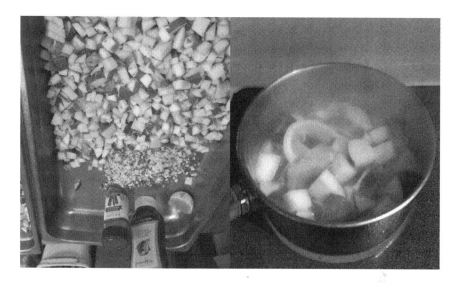

5. Chop fruit first, whether making apple cinnamon salad, apple kale salad or starting fruit sauce. If making sauce place fruit in a pot with water, cover fruit ½ way. Cook on stove medium high about 10 minutes until fork tender, let cool

30- minute mark

6. Clean and prep garlic. *save skins of onions and garlic for bone broth.

7. Chop and sauté onions, for everything

8. Start marinara by squishing tomatoes, putting some sautéed onions and olive oil in a pot. See recipe page 105.

9. Stuff the Stove Top, start cooking marinara, beans and quinoa.

See recipe page 107

60- minute mark

10. Season and tossy tossy your veggies for either roasting or grilling your choice. See recipe page 110

11. Dice and prep veggies, herbs, and flavors. These are the veggies you want to have recipe-ready when you like diced tomato, cucumber, and peppers. See recipe page 116

12. Work out proteins. If you are making meatloaf, balls, or burgers, it all starts the same way. Grab a bowl and the recipe on page 113.

13. Stuff The Oven. If you're roasting chicken, baking potatoes, making a meat loaf, or roasting veggies, get everything ready to cook at the same time. See recipe page 110

14. Fully sanitize counter, board, and knife

15. Check on things in the oven, and when items are fork tender, remove.

16. It's Blender Time Make protein pancake batter. See recipe page 122

17. Make mayo or salsa or salad dressing of the week (or anything else that requires a blender). See recipe page 120-121

18. Clean and put away the blender.

19. Chill marinara or beans in an ice bath.

20. Steam veggie selections, broccoli, spaghetti squash whole, beets, cabbage, etc. See recipe page 116

21. Cook pasta. See recipe page 109

22. Make compound butter or any other flavor set-ups. See recipe page 119

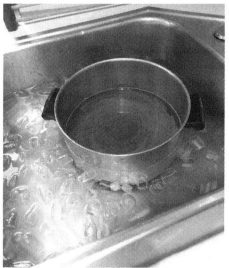

23. Pack-up food, marinate beef or chicken. *** Note: marinating just gets better and better the longer it sits. I like to marinate a minimum of 5 days, but you can go 7-8 days easy. Marinating is natural preserving at its best.

CHAPTER EIGHTEEN
RECIPES, TERMS AND TECHNIQUES

Okay, let's face it: our ancestors managed to figure this out without timers, thermometers, or iPhones, and you can too. Just pay attention and follow my lead.

Here are couple of techniques to learn

Tenderizing Meat. This little tool does the trick. Season your meat first, you are pushing the salt and flavor into your protein. This is THE way to tenderize leaner cuts of grass fed beef and make them tender.... Like butter! Tenderizing and marinated meat needs to rest for at least 1 day and up to 5 days.

Great marinades are everywhere. Last week's salad dressing, old juices, fresh garlic, even organic soy sauce with orange zest. Pretty much anything goes… except fresh ginger. The enzymes from ginger are so intense they will turn your meat fibers into mush.

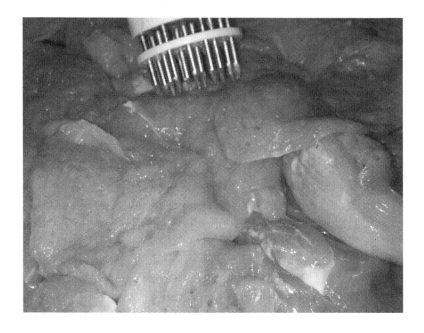

Toasting, Pounding and Grinding Spices – This is worth the work, the flavor pop is incredible.

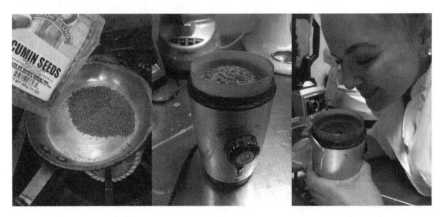

Toasting your spices add a whole new level of explosive flavor. I have a coffee grinder specifically for spices in my kitchen. And for those who need to blow off a bit if steam, pound peppercorns is just the task. I really like big hunk of peppercorns, but the more you pound, the smaller they become.

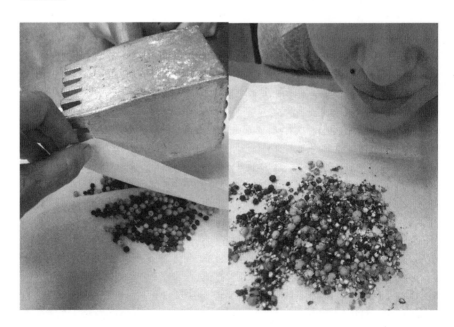

Cooking Garlic the right way.

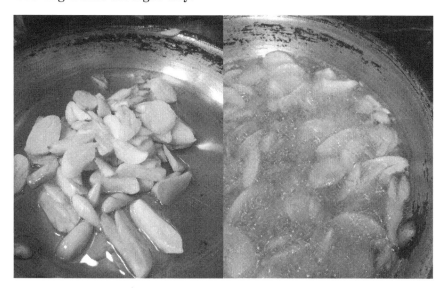

Start your pan cold. Yes you heard me correctly, start your pan cold with olive oil and garlic. Cook on medium high until the color develops around the edges and then remove from the pan to stop the cooking.

Adding raw minced garlic during the last minute or two of cooking is the trick for Asian food too. Garlic is meant to be gently cooked or raw. Burnt garlic is bitter and no fun.

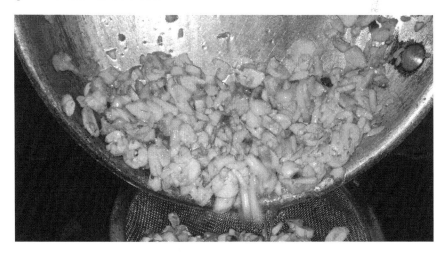

Fond is the maximum yummy bits on the bottom of the pan. Meat, onion, tomatoes, everything you cook when it browns created fond. Chefs around the world stay up at night dreaming of ways to create fond flavor. So Be fond to your fond! Take some water, pour into the pan and watch the show. Those delightful little bits you though were burnt on come right off and they are freaking delicious. Plus, then the pan is easy to wash ☺

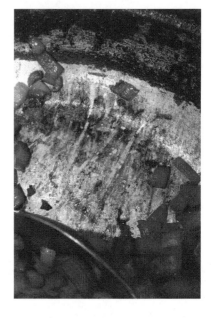

Tomato paste fond is great for developing flavor on a quick sauce!

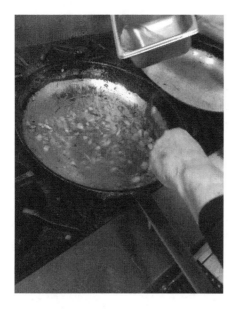

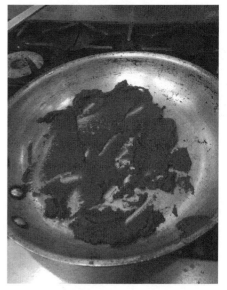

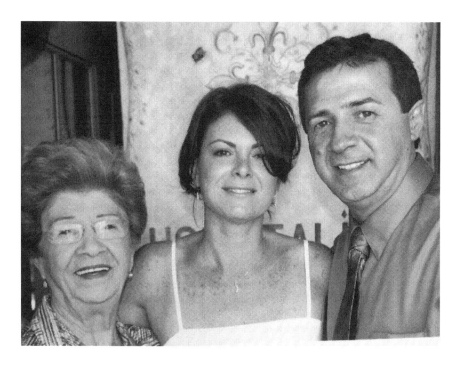

Mama, Rose Anthony Antonello

Mama Marinara Recipe

I learned this recipe from the Antonello Family. Theirs was the first kitchen I shared space in. I was serving Dan Marino at the time and the whole family loved the Antonellos' food. One day when Mama was making the marinara, I asked if I could learn and she lovingly said, "Hella no!" After endless nagging and persistence, she lovingly guided me through the recipe and its nuances. So here it is, reduced to a smaller batch size for you:

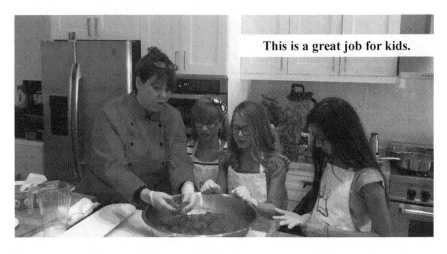

This is a great job for kids.

4 16oz cans of Italian plum tomatoes. Tomatoes squished and broken into little pieces, by hand.

4 large onions, chopped fine. You can use a food processor or blender. (*Save skins for bone broth)

1 cup of olive oil

½ cup dried basil

¼ cup dried oregano

Salt and pepper to taste

2 heads of garlic, chopped fine. Keep separate from onions.

Here's how to quickly peel your garlic (** Save skins for bone broth):

Add onions and oil into a large pot. Cook onions on medium high until translucent, not browned. Add in the herbs, salt, and pepper and cook for a few minutes to open up the flavor of the herbs. Then lastly add the garlic and continue to cook for only about 2 minutes and then add the plum tomatoes. Continue to cook on medium-high, stirring frequently as to not burn the bottom of the sauce, then reduce to a simmer. Cook for 2 hours and then cool in an ice bath. Freeze in containers you'll use in a week. Zip lock bags also work great.

*If storing in plastic freezer bags make sure to freeze on paper and a sheet pan. That way it won't get frozen into a funky shape that's stuck in the rungs of your wrack or on other products in your freezer.

Beans, Grains and Pasta
Beans
1lb beans
1 qt or so of water
½ tablespoon salt to taste
1 bay leaf
1 teas of baking soda

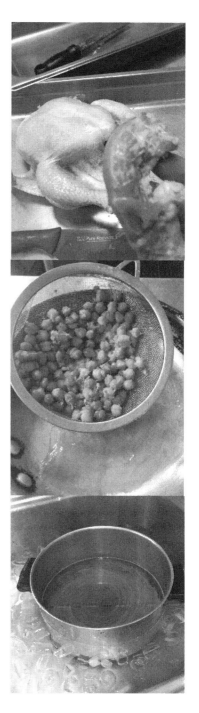

Chicken neck or wing from the whole chicken. Chicken bones add collagen and fats that make your beans silky and delicious.

Add anything else you love… garlic, onions, carrots. Just stay away from dominant flavors like curry or cumin. Keeping them plain now gives you more options at Jiffy Pan time.

Toss the beans on some baking paper and give a quick scan for stones or dirt. Pour them into our pot, add salt, bay leaf and baking soda. Cover with 4 inches or so of water and place on the burner, medium-high, and simmer about 90 minutes until beans are fork tender. Start checking 1 hour into cooking. Keep beans covered in water throughout the cooking and cooling processes, so add water when you need to.

Cool in an ice bath in your sink

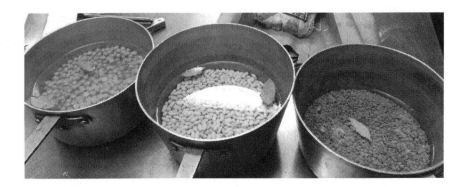

Grains

Almost all grains require a 2 to 1 ratio, meaning 2-parts water to 1-part grain. There are a few exceptions to this rule, such as black wild rice and polenta, so still read the instructions until you've memorized it. Beans and grains cook as they hydrate and soak up the liquid. It's important to start on high and let everything come to an active boil and then reduce to a simmer until they are fully cooked. Most grains cook for 20 minutes, but some thicker, more fibrous grains take as long as 40 minutes.

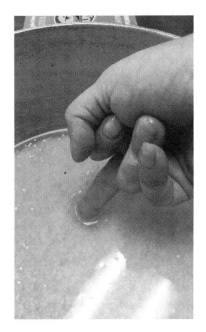

For a quick measure on 2 to 1 ratio grains, such as rice and quinoa, just give the finger! Yep, pour the grain in a pot and add water up to your middle finger's first knuckle. This works every time. Also, you can always add extra water in the beginning and then strain off excess after 20 minutes of cooking.

Quinoa is a 2 to 1 ratio cook. The important thing with quinoa is to soak the grains about 20 minutes, drain off liquid, then add what you need back in. Quinoa's outer shell is bitter and can soaked and drained off.

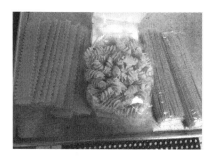

Pasta. I know you already know how to boil up some pasta. But if you really like it and want to cook off two different shapes, you can cook them in the same pot at the same time. Check the cook times on each, add the one that cooks the longest first, wait the few minutes' difference, and then add the second shape so they both finish at the same time. Also, undercook pasta by 1 minute for al dente so you don't overcook come Jiffy Pan time.

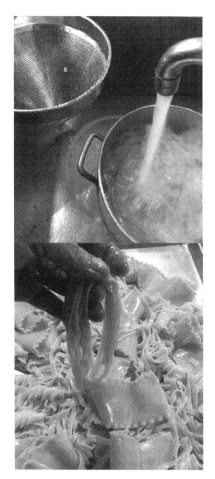

Drain off pasta, add cold water back into your pot, and add pasta back in. This helps removes startches and allows you to precook your pasta with out the sticking problem. *By cooking the pasta al dente and rinsing off excess starches it raises the glymic index less ☺

Let rest a minute or two in cold water and drain again.

And then pour off into a bowl or onto a sheet pan, drizzle with olive oil, then separate. It's important to know this works great with pastas that are very different in shape and size.

Roasting 101

Set oven to bake at 375 or convection bake 350 degrees, that's roasting. Simple.

Whole chicken – chicken bone broth, Jewish penicillin

Roasting a whole chicken is super easy: Get your baking pan. Open your chicken in baking pan. To wash or not to wash your poultry? I say no. Salt is sanitizing and letting it develop by resting is the ticket! Plus, you don't run the risk of cross-contaminating your whole kitchen.

Season your chicken inside and out with whatever you love. Salt, pepper, lemon, lime or orange zest, garlic, rosemary… you get the idea. *But no fresh ginger on meats, ever! Why no ginger? Fresh ginger is so rich in enzymes it can turn your raw or cooked meat to mush in a couple of days.

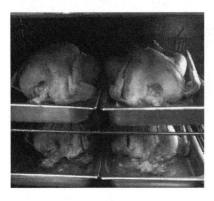

Rub the season into the meat. The trick is to let the seasoning rest on the meat for about 20 minutes and rub again before you place it in the oven.

Bake at roasting temperature, 375 degrees, until the skin is golden brown. As soon as it's that perfect color of golden brown, 'bout an hour, use your meat thermometer to check the internal temp. Stick in the meaty part of the thigh, midway and you want 160 degrees. The bird will continue to cook and get to 165 even when it's removed from the oven. Let it rest and cool. If you're cooking to serve immediately, still let the chicken rest for 30 minutes before carving.

For your bone broth or gravy:

When your bird is cooled down, remove it from the pan. Next add about two cups of hot water to the baking pan and scrape up all the drippings, the goodies and bits on the bottom of the pan. Pour into a jar until you're ready to make the bone broth. This is the stuff French chefs dream about at night.

You can carve off the bone for many meals. When you have eaten the meat, save the bones and skin for your bone broth. On your next meal prep day pop them in the oven until golden brown.

Chicken Bone Broth

1 chicken carcass = 1 gallon of bone broth
Bake the empty carcass and skins for about 30 minute. Add the browned bones and reserved fond broth you saved when you first cooked the chicken. Add water, the reserved onion and garlic skins, salt and bay leave. Simmer, don't boil for 1 to 2 hours. If you are short on freezer space, make your own concentrate by simmering down to 1 quart of broth from 1 gallon. Then when serving, add water to correct proportion.

To make the broth, roast the bones again or put directly into 1 gallon of water with

Onion & garlic skins

Carrots

Bay leave

Sea salt with minerals

Boil for about 2 hours, strain and cool in an ice bathy.

The ice bath trick is so awesome because it will cool any sauce or stock down to chilly in just 15 minutes. Stir often.

*It's very important too cool down all of your food before packing and placing your fridge. This step will increase your shelf life and prevent you from blowing out the cold temperature in your fridge when loading it up with freshly made food.

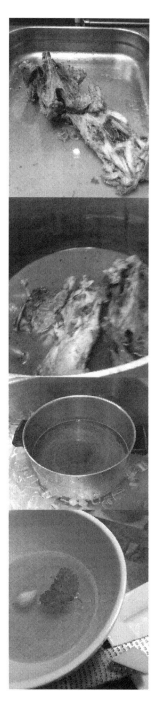

Roasting Veggies. Same rules of seasoning and resting and then cooking until you have color appeal apply. I typically cook at 400 degrees. Always check for knife tender consistency for doneness.

Tossy tossy is one of my favorite ways to distribute seasoning and oil onto your veggies.

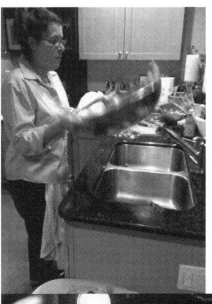

An easy way to deal with different bake times on the same sheet pan is to cut baking paper into sections so you can remove specific items you want, when you want with ease. When roasting check on the items in your oven every 30 minutes, minimum.

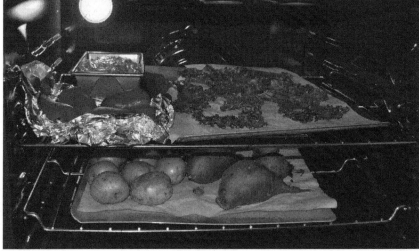

Ground Meat options: balls, loaf, and patties

Base recipe for balls, loaf, and patties

1lb of ground meat, beef, chicken or turkey

1 egg

¼ cup ground oatmeal or organic bread crumbs

½ cup of sautéed onions

½ cup of moist flavor of your choice. Examples include, tomato paste, salsa, marinara, low sugar ketchup or BBQ sauce, teriyaki sauce, chimichurri sauce, basil spinach pesto, mojo, salad dressing, fruit sauce, honey, mustard, fresh herbs, dried herbs, and chopped cooked bacon... you get the idea. One of my favorite combos for guys is tomato paste and pounded pepper corns. The Lycopene in the tomato paste is a huge boost for the prostate gland.

*I like to mix dark and light ground turkey for a lighter yet still delicious blend.

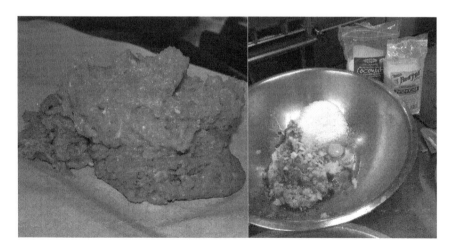

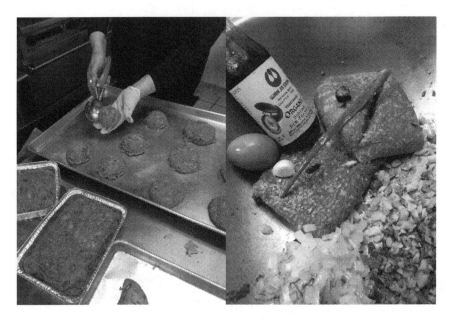

Now you can form into balls, a loaf, or patties and roast or grill. I love my scoops for portioning out my protein. It's a big time saver.

Note* If grilling grass-fed beef, add 1 extra yolk to mix to keep patties from breaking apart when cooking. And giving them a quick spray of non-stick spray does the trick. I really like this spectrum, product

Sautéed Ground meat in dishes such as chili, taco meat, Bolognese meat sauce, or Thai peanut chicken, for examples. I cook using the similar technique. Beef, chicken, or turkey all work the same. Forget about pouring oil in and then draining it off and throwing it away. Start with a dry pan, yes no oil for the meat, instead use the oil to toast and open up the flavor of your seasonings.

Have all of your ingredients ready before starting this dish. Add meat to pre-heated sauté pan, no oil. Yep I really just said no oil, yet. Tip your pan and add oil and your herbs and spices, then stir the spices in the oil to open up their flavors and then fold into the un-browned meat.

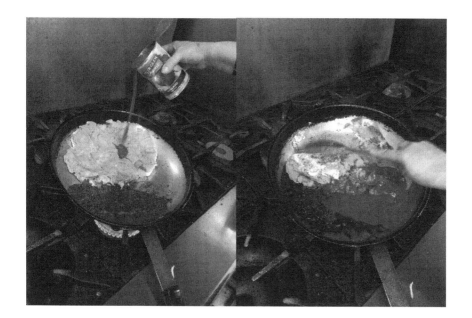

Brown the bottom of the meat, but you can leave the rest still uncooked as you add your liquid sauce, whether tomato sauce for chili or peanut sauce for Thai or your marsala wine for ground chicken marsala… you get the idea. The French call that brown stuck on meat and flavor at the bottom of the pan "fond". Be fond to your fond. The liquid will loosen the stuck meat off the pan, still giving you that deep brown flavor, but the uncooked meat will simply breakdown without the fight of fully browning the meat first.

Marinated Chicken or beef

Marinating chicken breasts, steak and other large cuts of meat is a great way to tenderize and flavor up your protein. Marinating is most amazing when you've given your meat 4 to 5 days to soak up the love.

Steamed Veggies

Here's the thing: food continues to cook for a short time after it is removed from the heat, and this is especially true for steaming. So to save the step of putting things in ice after removing from the steamer, I just cook for a little less time and let it cook through while resting. I get great color results and I have one less thing to wash. Here's my base time schedule for steaming veggies:

Broccoli 1 minute

Green beans 2 minutes

Carrots 5 minutes

Chopped Veggies, fermented cabbage, salads and salsas 101:

A sharp knife, a mandolin, and skills make this quick work.

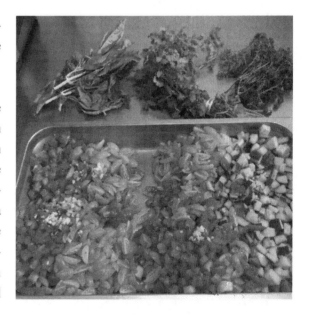

From the items on the left, I can make fresh salsa, tomato, onion cilantro or I can make tomato, onion and garlic Italian bruschetta or Israeli salad. Store your cut veggies separatly if for maximum flexibility at meal time.

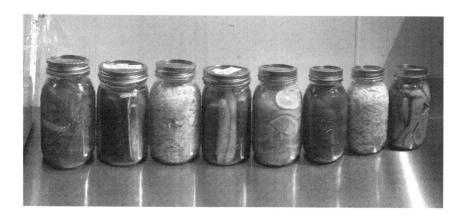

Fermented Cabbage This is really a must-eat food for all in my opinion. I'm a big believer in eating just a few bites with every meal you eat. And you can drink the brine too, as I often do first thing in the morning, especially if I've torn up my gut lining from catering food and stress the night before. Fermented cabbage carries the full spectrum of prebiotic and probiotic strains that naturally work every time for you.

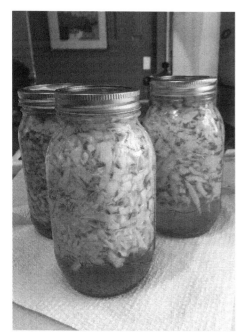

1 head of cabbage, red or white

1 tablespoon salt

¼ cup of caraway seeds, or dill seed, fennel seeds, fresh dill, garlic, onion, lemon slices, lime slices, orange slices, you get the idea.

You can ferment pretty much anything too, not just cabbage. Veggies that have a high water content like bok choy, peppers, and onions don't hold their texture and become very soft.

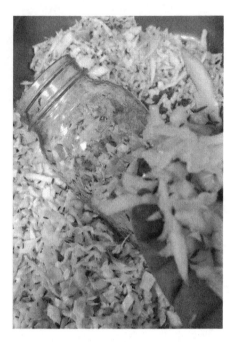

Chop up the cabbage, sprinkle and toss with salt and caraway. Fill jars with the cabbage 1 inch from the top. This is important because the fermentation process needs room to build; if not, you run the risk of your fermentation over-flowing the jar. That's why I place my jars in the sink or on a paper towel until ready.

Let ferment on the counter 36 to 48 hours. Then you'll see a tiny bubble when you jiggle the jars. Now this is very important: when you open your jars for the first time, open over the sink. The fermentation causes carbonation and it will explode a little when you open it.

I'm often asked if it needs to be refrigerated after opening and the answer is, "yes". And that's because our ancestors found the alien time portal Captain Kirk and Spock left unlocked and they traveled back and forth putting their fermented cabbage into random refrigerators. Ok, so the correct answer is no. It never goes bad folks, it just continues to build probiotics. ***just make sure your cabbage is always covered with brine. You can add more water if you need to.

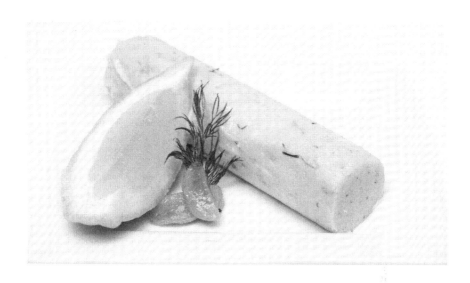

Fats and Flavors

Compound organic butters. These are so much fun to serve as a spread or for cooking.

Soften butter by leaving out on the counter for a few hours. Add any combination of herbs and spices you love. Here are a few ideas:

Smoked peppercorn, pounded peppercorns, liquid smoke

Smoked herb, with scallions, basil and liquid smoke

Citrus honey with fresh citrus zest either lemon, orange or honey

Maple butter with maple syrup and maple extract

Roasted red pepper and even sautéed onions left over from other dishes

make great flavors *Don't waste the grace ☺

Pesto's are another fantastic place to put citrus zest, fresh herbs, nuts and cheeses if you wish. I like to keep the cheese out of my pesto's to keep them more versatile for sautéing veggies or drizzling on top of carbs or protein. Cheese in pesto's tend to burn on the bottom of pans and feel sad for the waste.

Salad dressing

The base recipe for most every dressing is as follows:

1 egg yolk or 2 tablespoons of mustard or 2 tablespoons of honey.

1/2 cup vinegar, red, white, or balsamic.

Blend and slowly add 1 cup of oil and finish with a ¼ cup of water.

From here you can add anything you wish such as

Salt, truffle salt, smoked salt, roasted veggies, roasted peppers, pounded pepper corns, grilled onions, fresh basil, fresh cilantro, spinach, avocado, tomatoes…. Well, you get the idea. Last week's dressing makes a great marinate for this week. Salad dressing can freeze for later use at a marinade.
*Don't waste the grace ☺

Mayonnaise

1 egg yolk- add leftover white to meatloaf mix or protein pancake mix.

1/2 teaspoon season salt

1/2 teaspoon dry mustard

1 cup oil of expeller press grapeseed oil, organic canola oil or olive oil

1/8 teas sugar

2 teaspoons fresh squeezed lemon juice

1 tablespoon white wine vinegar

Add the yolks and mustard to the blender, slowly add oil in a very thin stream until thick. Add salt, sugar, lemon juice, and vinegar in the blender. Continue to blend to incorporate. Will last 1 week in the fridge. You can split this recipe in half and whisk by hand

Applesauce or fruit sauce and baby food. Place chopped apples, pears, or any fruit you like in a sauce pan, add about 2 inches of water to the pan, and top with a lid. Place on medium-high and cook for 10 minutes until your fruit is knife tender. Remove from burner, let cook. When cooled, place only the fruit in the blender and begin blending. See if you get the consistency you want with just the fruit; you can always add water but you can't remove it. If you add too much water and your sauce becomes thin, you can thicken by adding a banana or two. Save the fruit water, it's great to drink warm or chilled.

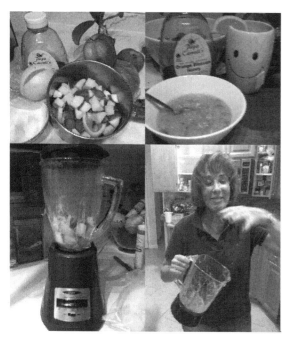

Homemade apple sauce is so delicious this student licked the blender and her fingers as to not throw a drop away. It's that good!

If you're making baby food your two goals are puree the cooked veggies or fruits and strain to remove any stringy long fibers that your baby can't chew due to the lack of the teeth. That's it folks, it's that easy!

*Note when introducing foods to your baby, consult with your pediatrician and start foods one at a time. No, mixing squash and apples at first.

I'm hearing that song. I hear it is folks, "Anything they can make you can make better, anything they can sell you can make fresher, yes you can!!! I'm putting this recipe in because of my recent trip to grocery store and finding manufacturers are shifting away from glass and now putting baby food in the plastic squeezy bottles. There are better options for our babies.

Frozen Fruit Pops! Your fruit sauces are exactly what you need to make frozen fruit pops too! Freeze your left overs for smoothies and protein drinks too. *Don't waste the grace ☺

Protein Pancakes. This recipe saves me for breakfast on the run, clients love'm (grown-up and kids alike), and they are perfect for when I'm craving carbs and just want to shove a hot sweet pancake in my mouth.

1 ½ cups of oatmeal

6 eggs

¾ cup of whey protein isolate

*optional

1 teaspoon baking soda

1 tablespoon molasses

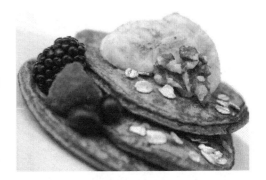

1 cup of moist fruit flavors of your choice. So bananas, blueberries, strawberries, apples, pears, peaches, mangos and all of the above will be D'licious.

1 cup of diced fruit & nuts to add in when cooking *optional

Blend everything the blender. Start with oats and grind them up, then add everything else. You can hold this batter and cook pancakes fresh all week. The batter will stay fresh in the fridge for 10 days. They cook just like regular pancakes. Whey protein isolates seem to work best. You can omit the protein at first, and then add a little to a couple of scoops of batter. Cook them to test if you your protein works well for texture. I like MRM ᵗᵐ and About Time ᵗᵐ for texture!

*protein drink

I like, ALL of the top athletes I know, start every day off with at least a cup of spinach stuffed into a protein drink. This is my daily diligence to start off my day with 2 serving of veggies! I put ice, water, protein powder, spinach and I like a little avocado too to make it creamy. Banana and mango a great to add too to change up the taste.

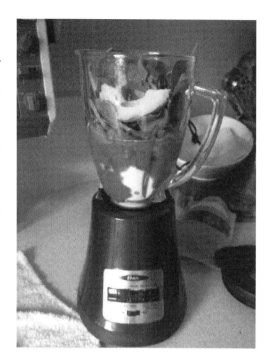

CHAPTER NINETEEN
YOUR REWARD AND JIFFY PAN TRICKS.

Now you have choices, choices, choices. So let's talk combinations now. Your fats and flavors items will dictate what you make. So any combination of the herbs, spices, dressings, and sauces are available to you. Let me show you the combinations:

Italian Marinara

Marinara + chicken + quinoa + veggies = Chicken Cacciatore Primavera

Marinara + cream = pink sauce

Pasta + garbanzo beans + zucchini + Marinara + vinegar and oil = Pasta Salad

Chicken bone broth + white beans + pasta + Marinara + rosemary = pasta e fagoile

Noodles + soy sauce, ginger, sesame seed oil = Asian

Fish sauce + cilantro + ginger + peanuts and or butter = Thai (Noodles)

(protein) (broccoli) (asparagus) (beans) (anything)

You get the idea now…. Go play with your food!

I recommend getting a jiffy pan for every member of your family if possible. I heat up everyone's wholesome meal just the way they want it in their own pan. Let's face it: for most families, the idea of everyone wanting to eat the same thing for dinner happens like, never. If your family is used to choosing, you can now offer Italian, Asian, French, Southern, Latin, or your own creations in 4 minutes.

I have two techniques to share:
One is Steam and Heat and the other is Sauté and Steam to heat

Steam and Heat

Heat 4 tablespoons of water to boiling. You'll have about two tablespoons left once hot, then place your food in the pan. Top with lid and turn to low for 3 minutes and turn burner off. In this time, the scant 2 tablespoons water will be cooked off. You can play with this amount, especially if you're heating up something thirsty like mashed potatoes. You can leave your pan on the warm burner until you are ready. I like to call this carryover heat and I use it a lot, plus you can't ever burn your meal this way.

If you're cooking for two and you both want the same foods, this trick works great in large sauté pans too. I recommend you double the water to ½ cup. Start on high for 1 minutes and leave to simmer for 5 minutes, turn off the burner, and let rest until you're ready. Remove lid and serve.

Sauté and Steam

Start with your oil and/or butter and sauté your onions or whatever veggies or protein you like freshly cooked. When you get your desired brownness, add everything else to your pan, grab your lid. Pour ¼ water into the pan and quickly top the pan with the lid to capture the steam. Cook on high for 30 seconds.

CHAPTER TWENTY
SNACKING AND SUGAR CRUSHERS!

What crushes a sweet craving???

Protein and Fats. That's why I love the protein pancake recipe and Snack Bites. Evening snacking is the witching hour for us sugar junkies. And God help me if I'm watching live TV and need to suffer through the ridiculous food commercials.

I eat frozen grapes and homemade fruit pops to help ease the cravings.

Another technique I use and suggest is emotional freedom tapping. My favorite video is from Gabby Bernstein, Spirit Junkie, at https://www.youtube.com/watch?v=I6djaQz-0Gs

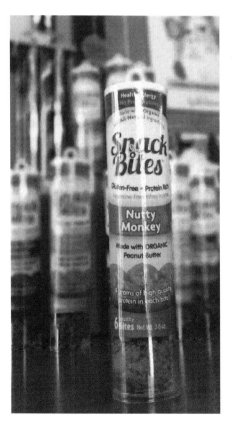

But eating protein and fats is truly the most efficient way to break the sugar habit. How many snack bite flavors does it take to lose 80 pounds, well for me it's been six! How do you know they taste good?

Snack Bites are an Awarding winning celebrity chef created snack.

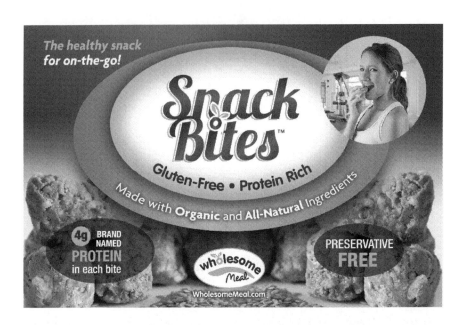

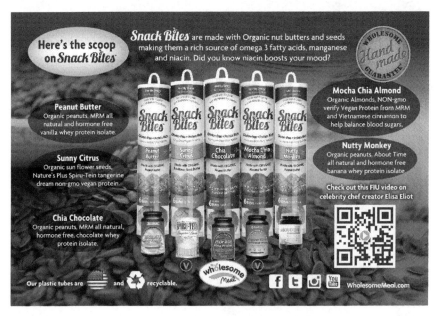

128

Let's stay in touch.

Join my e-newsletter at **www.wholesomemeal.com**

Thank you for your time. I hope you find what you learned simple and easy to remember for your healthful journey.

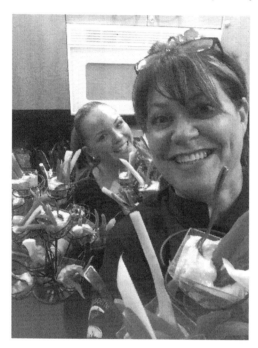

A special shout out to Lauren Sepulvida, every day I appreciate what you bring to my day & the art.

Twitter: Wholesome Meal@wholesomemeal

Snack Bites@Snackbites4you

www.facebook.com/WholesomeMealSnackBites

www.facebook.com/ChefElisaCatering

Instagram: Wholesomemeal and Snackbites

www.chefeliscatering.com

RESOURCE PAGES

Harvard 20 year study of 100,000 participant proving the reduced risk of chronic diseases in those that ate a nutrient dense diet
http://www.ncbi.nlm.nih.gov/pubmed/21496749

Wholefoods ANDI Score

Understanding Saturated Fat
http://linkis.com/huffingtonpost.com/q83FY
www.youtube.com/watch?v=IQlNv2Au-Lg
http://archinte.jamanetwork.com/article.aspx?articleid=2173094 (health benefits of peanuts)
http://bit.ly/1DwyIVo
http://en.wikipedia.org/wiki/Epidemiology_of_autism
http://www.huffingtonpost.com/2014/10/06/breakfast-most-important-history_n_5910054.html
http://www.autism-society.org/what-is/facts-and-statistics/
Prevalence in the United States is estimated at 1 in 68 births. (CDC, 2014)
http://www.autism-society.org/what-is/facts-and-statistics/
More than 3.5 million Americans live with an autism spectrum disorder. (Buescher et al., 2014)
Prevalence of autism in U.S. children increased by 119.4 percent from 2000 (1 in 150) to 2010 (1 in 68). (CDC, 2014) Autism is the fastest-growing developmental disability. (CDC, 2008)
1,794 drugs recalled between 2004 and 2011
http://abcnews.go.com/blogs/health/2012/06/04/u-s-has-drug-recall-problem-study-says/
Epidemiology of autism
From Wikipedia, the free encyclopedia

The epidemiology of autism is the study of factors affecting autism spectrum disorders (ASD). A 2012 review of global prevalence estimates of autism spectrum disorders found a median of 62 cases per 10,000 people. [1] There is a lack of evidence from low- and middle-income countries though.[1]

ASD averages a 4.3:1 male-to-female ratio.[2] The number of children known to have autism has increased dramatically since the 1980s, at least partly due to changes in diagnostic practice; it is unclear whether prevalence has actually increased;[2] and as-yet-unidentified environmental risk factors cannot be ruled out.[3] The risk of autism is associated with several prenatal factors, including advanced parental age and diabetes in the mother during pregnancy.[4] ASD is associated with several genetic disorders[5] and with epilepsy.[6]

Coeliac disease (/'siːli.æk/; celiac disease in the United States[1] and often celiac sprue) is an autoimmune disorder of the small intestine that occurs in genetically predisposed people of all ages from middle infancy onward. Symptoms include pain and discomfort in the digestive tract, chronic constipation and diarrhoea, failure to thrive (in children), anaemia[2] and fatigue, but these may be absent, and symptoms in other organ systems have been described. Vitamin deficiencies are often noted in people with coeliac disease owing to the reduced ability of the small intestine to properly absorb nutrients from food.
http://www.ncbi.nlm.nih.gov/pmc/articles/PMC27435/. *Inflammation and nutrition upload*
http://www.livestrong.com/article/198975-what-are-the-dangers-of-palm-oil/

In a 2005 report entitled "Cruel Oil: How Palm Oil Harms Health, Rainforest & Wildlife," the Center for Science in the Public Interest concedes that palm oil is less harmful than partially hydrogenated soybean oil, but it points out that it "is still considerably less healthful than other vegetable oils." In support of its warnings about the dangers of palm oil, the center cites two meta-analyses that show that palm oil raises blood cholesterol levels. A 1997 British analysis evaluated 147 human trials and concluded that palmitic acid, an active ingredient in palm oil, raised total blood cholesterol levels. A Dutch analysis, released in 2003, weighed data from 35 clinical studies and found that palmitic acid significantly increased the ratio of total cholesterol to so-called "good cholesterol," a widely recognized risk factor for heart disease.

Difficult to Digest

In "Cooking for Healthy Healing," author Linda Page, Ph.D., a naturopathic practitioner, acknowledges some of the health benefits of palm oil but notes that it is very difficult to get palm oil that hasn't been heavily refined. The refining process depletes many of the nutrients that occur naturally in the oil and also makes the oil much more difficult to digest. For these reasons, Page recommends that palm oil be avoided.
http://www.nufarm.com/assets/26570/1/Omega-3collaborationupdatere-leaseJan2014Final.pdf?download
http://www.bloomberg.com/news/articles/2012-10-11/asian-seafood-raised-on-pig-feces-approved-for-u-s-consumers
http://circ.ahajournals.org/content/120/11/1011.full.pdf 100 sugar calories for women, 150 for menuhttp://healthyamericans.org/obesity/ for rates tripling.
http://www.mayoclinic.org/healthy-lifestyle/nutrition-and-healthy-eating/expert-answers/bpa/faq-20058331 BPA warning
http://www.motherjones.com/environment/2014/03/tritan-certichem-eastman-bpa-free-plastic-safe
http://www.mdtmag.com/news/2013/07/sugar-makes-cancer-light-mri-scanners?et_cid=3355921&et_rid=413500061&type=cta#.Udr5P-Ar98t
http://www.npr.org/sections/health-shots/2014/09/05/345534115/science-on-diets-is-low-in-essential-information
https://www.sciencebasedmedicine.org/microwaves-and-nutrition/

Made in United States
Orlando, FL
20 November 2021

10564201R00085